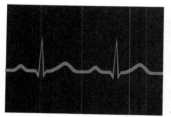

Combatting Cardiovascular Diseases Skillfully

SECOND EDITION
NURSING84 BOOKS™
SPRINGHOUSE CORPORATION
SPRINGHOUSE, PENNSYLVANIA

NURSING84 BOOKS™

NEW NURSING SKILLBOOK™ SERIES
Giving Emergency Care Competently
Monitoring Fluid and Electrolytes Precisely
Assessing Vital Functions Accurately
Coping with Neurologic Problems Proficiently
Reading EKGs Correctly
Combatting Cardiovascular Diseases Skillfully
Nursing Critically Ill Patients Confidently
Dealing with Death and Dying

NURSING PHOTOBOOK™ SERIES
Providing Respiratory Care
Managing I.V. Therapy
Dealing with Emergencies
Giving Medications
Assessing Your Patients
Using Monitors
Providing Early Mobility
Giving Cardiac Care
Performing GI Procedures
Implementing Urologic Procedures
Controlling Infection
Ensuring Intensive Care
Coping with Neurologic Disorders
Caring for Surgical Patients
Working with Orthopedic Patients
Nursing Pediatric Patients
Helping Geriatric Patients
Attending Ob/Gyn Patients
Aiding Ambulatory Patients
Carrying Out Special Procedures

NURSE'S REFERENCE LIBRARY®
Diseases
Diagnostics
Drugs
Assessment
Procedures
Definitions
Practices
Emergencies

NURSING NOW™
Shock
Hypertension
Drug Interactions
Cardiac Crises
Respiratory Emergencies
Pain

NURSE'S CLINICAL LIBRARY™
Cardiovascular Disorders
Respiratory Disorders
Endocrine Disorders
Neurologic Disorders
Renal and Urologic Disorders

Nursing84 DRUG HANDBOOK™

Combatting
Cardiovascular Diseases
Skillfully

NEW NURSING SKILLBOOK™
Series
PROGRAM DIRECTOR
Jean Robinson

CLINICAL DIRECTOR
Barbara McVan, RN

PROJECT MANAGER
Susan Rossi Williams

**Springhouse Corporation
Book Division**
CHAIRMAN
Eugene W. Jackson

PRESIDENT
Daniel L. Cheney

VICE-PRESIDENT AND
DIRECTOR
Timothy B. King

VICE-PRESIDENT, BOOK
OPERATIONS
Thomas A. Temple

VICE-PRESIDENT, PRODUCTION
AND PURCHASING
Bacil Guiley

RESEARCH DIRECTOR
Elizabeth O'Brien

Staff for first edition:
BOOK EDITOR: Helen Hamilton
CLINICAL EDITORS: Catherine Manzi, RN; Minnie Rose, RN, BSN, MEd
MARGINALIA EDITOR: Avery Rome
COPY EDITOR: Patricia Hamilton
RESEARCHER AND INDEXER: Vonda Heller
PRODUCTION MANAGER: Bernard Haas
TYPOGRAPHY MANAGER: David C. Kosten
PRODUCTION ASSISTANT: Betty Mancini
DESIGNER: Maggie Arnott
ARTISTS: Robert Goldstein, Robert Jackson, Robert H. Renn, Sandra Simms
Cover and divider art by Robert Goldstein

Clinical consultants for first edition:
Kathleen Dracup, BSN, MN, *Clinical Professor, University of California at Los Angeles School of Nursing*
Peter G. Lavine, MD, *Director of Coronary Care Unit, Crozer-Chester Medical Center, Chester, Pa.*
Despina Seremelis, RN, BSN, *Staff Nurse, Temple University Hospital, Philadelphia*

Staff for this edition:
BOOK EDITOR: Patricia R. Urosevich
CLINICAL EDITOR: Barbara McVan, RN
ASSISTANT EDITOR: Jo Lennon
DESIGNER: Kathaleen Motak Singel
COPY SUPERVISOR: David R. Moreau
COPY EDITOR: Diane M. Labus
EDITORIAL STAFF ASSISTANT: Ellen Johnson
ART PRODUCTION MANAGER: Robert Perry
ARTISTS: Diane Fox, Donald G. Knauss, Robert Miele, Sandra Sanders, Louise Stamper, Robert Wieder
TYPOGRAPHY MANAGER: David C. Kosten
TYPOGRAPHY ASSISTANTS: Ethel Halle, Diane Paluba, Nancy Wirs
PRODUCTION MANAGER: Wilbur D. Davidson
COVER ART: Robert Jackson
COVER PHOTO: Paul Cohen
DIVIDER ART: Robert Goldstein

Clinical consultants for this edition:
Robert Biern, MD, *Director, Coronary Care Unit and Heart Station, Anne Arundel General Hospital, Annapolis, Md.*
Mary L. Clements, RN, *Relief Charge Nurse, Northampton—Accomack Memorial Hospital, Nassawadox, Va.*
Kathleen M. McCauley, RN, BSN, MSN, *Cardiovascular Clinical Specialist, Hospital of the University of Pennsylvania; Clinical Instructor, University of Pennsylvania School of Nursing, Philadelphia*

Library of Congress Cataloging in Publication Data

Main entry under title:

Combatting cardiovascular diseases skillfully.
  (New Nursing Skillbook series)
  "Nursing84 books."
  Bibliography: p.
  Includes index.
  1. Cardiovascular disease nursing. I. Series: New nursing skillbook. [DNLM:
1. Cardiovascular diseases—Nursing. WY 152.2 C729]

RC674.C63 1984
616.1'2'0024613   84-563
ISBN 0-916730-66-2

Contents

Contributors

Sally A. Bowers, a graduate of Johns Hopkins Hospital School of Nursing, is a staff nurse in the cardiovascular intensive care unit, Toronto Western Hospital. She completed a training program in coronary care at the University of Maryland, Baltimore.

Christine Sue Breu has a BSN degree from Marian College of Fond du Lac in Michigan. She has an MN degree from the University of California at Los Angeles School of Nursing, where she is an assistant clinical instructor.

Marie Scott Brown is an associate professor of parent-child nursing at the University of Colorado School of Nursing, where she earned MSN, MA, and PhD degrees. She is a BSN degree graduate of Marquette University, Milwaukee. She is a member of the National Association for Pediatric Nurse Associates and Practitioners.

Christine W. Cannon has a BS degree from the University of Pennsylvania, Philadelphia. She is a medical clinical specialist at Wilmington (Del.) Medical Center. She belongs to the American Association of Critical-Care Nurses and Sigma Theta Tau.

Mary M. Canobbio is a nurse-teacher-practitioner at Kaiser Permanente Medical Center, Los Angeles. An AA degree graduate of Los Angeles City College, Department of Nursing, she earned her BSN degree at California State University, Los Angeles.

Kathleen A. Dracup, an advisor on this book, is an assistant clinical professor at the University of California at Los Angeles School of Nursing, where she also earned her MN degree. She has a BSN degree from St. Xavier's College, Chicago.

Lauren Marie Isacson graduated from the Ann May School of Nursing, Jersey Shore Medical Center, Neptune, New Jersey, where she is a nursing education instructor.

Gail D'Onofrio Long has a BS degree from Duke University, Durham, North Carolina, and an MS degree from Boston University, where she is a clinical specialist in the medical intensive/coronary care units. She has a certificate in advanced life support.

Rosemary Jarlath Maloney is a clinical nurse at Tripler Army Medical Center, Honolulu. She has a BSN degree from Gwynedd Mercy College, Springhouse, Pennsylvania, and an MSN degree from the University of Pennsylvania, Philadelphia.

Catherine Ciaverelli Manzi graduated from Hahnemann Hospital School of Nursing, Philadelphia. She was head nurse of the cardiac intensive care center at Hahnemann Medical College and Hospital. She was a clinical editor for the original Nursing Skillbook series.

Kathy Murphy is nursing program coordinator at the University of Maine, Fort Kent. She received her BSN degree from the University of Maine, Portland, and her MSN degree from the University of Pennsylvania School of Nursing, Philadelphia. She's working toward a PhD at New York (N.Y.) University.

Mary Alexander Murphy has BSN and MS degrees and a nurse practitioner certificate from the University of Colorado, Denver, where she is an instructor in the school of medicine, department of pediatrics. She is a doctoral candidate at the University of Denver.

Idabelle Ream, a diploma graduate of Philadelphia General Hospital, is system coordinator at Hahnemann University Hospital, Philadelphia, and a member of the American Association of Critical-Care Nurses.

Minnie Bowen Rose has a BSN degree from Indiana University, Bloomington, and an MEd degree from Temple University, Philadelphia. She was a clinical editor for the original Nursing Skillbook series.

Klaus J. Schulz has an MD degree from Freie Universitat, Berlin. He is staff cardiologist and director of the pacemaker evaluation center at Jersey Shore Medical Center, Neptune, New Jersey.

Kit Stahler-Miller has BSN and MSN degrees from the University of Pennsylvania. She's an instructor in the Deparment of Nursing at La Salle College, Philadelphia.

Arlene B. Strong is a cardiac clinical specialist and an adult nurse practitioner in the anticoagulant clinic at the Veterans Administration Hospital, Portland, Oregon. She has a BSN degree from the University of Portland and an MN degree from the University of Oregon, Portland.

M. Sandy Wyper has BSN and MSN degrees from Case Western Reserve University, Cleveland, where she teaches medical-surgical nursing at Frances Payne Bolton School of Nursing. She is a member of the nursing honor society, Sigma Theta Tau.

Advisory Board

Foreword

Cardiovascular nursing no longer means just the care of patients in the coronary care unit. Besides direct nursing care, nurses are expected to promote health and prevent cardiovascular disease in many ways.

Technologic advances in diagnosis and treatment, sophisticated equipment, current trends toward early detection and prevention of risk factors, and increased emphasis on rehabilitation and patient teaching all have greatly expanded nurses' responsibilities to patients with cardiovascular disease. Nurses now screen patients for blood pressure abnormalities and give counseling about this and other risk factors. Many general staff nurses are responsible for preparing the cardiac patient through teaching and discharge planning. And public health nurses run community clinics designed to help people who need supervision during chronic illness.

To participate in health care in these important ways, you must have highly developed skills in physical assessment, history taking, diagnostic test interpretation, and health teaching. Your contribution through nursing assessment can hardly be overstated. Although you don't establish the patient's diagnosis, you must oversee his progress under treatment. No patient's condition remains static. In case of serious cardiovascular disease, improvement means a chance for survival; deterioration can mean sudden death. Unquestionably then, every patient with cardiovascular disease needs continuing assessment of his physiologic status and of his response to treatment. Such assessment is primarily a nursing task, and the skills and enthusiasm you bring to this task profoundly influence the patient's survival.

This New Nursing Skillbook can help you review and update the skills you need to offer patients with cardiovascular disease the best possible care. Fully revised and up-to-the-minute, it begins with a brief review of pediatric cardiology (which includes congenital anomalies and their surgical correction). It continues with the most common forms of acquired cardiovascular disease in adults. This, the most comprehensive section of the book, includes a detailed review of physical assessment in adults; a summary of the most useful diagnostic studies, including how to prepare patients for these tests and how to understand their results; and in several chapters, a discussion of coronary artery disease in its various stages of severity. The same section includes chapters on how to recognize and deal with cardiomyopathy and inflammatory diseases of the heart. Other chapters in this fully updated section tell how to cope with cardiogenic shock, pulmonary edema, and pacemakers. The final section of this book deals briefly with the management of vascular disease, including peripheral vascular disease and aneurysms.

Throughout, this New Nursing Skillbook focuses on the nurse's role as a member of the health team. It lists what symptoms to expect and how to evaluate them; how to recognize important complications; how to plan, coordinate, and provide total care; how to provide psychological support; and how to help with rehabilitation. A nurse who does all of these things well can help restore the patient to his maximum potential.

All in all, this new edition of one of the most popular Skillbooks offers a handy reference. Mastering its contents can help you to improve your care of patients with cardiovascular disease and make you a more valuable member of the health-care team. Your resulting confidence in the quality of care you feel competent to give can only enhance your satisfaction in nursing.

—ROSE PINNEO, RN, MS
Associate Professor of Nursing and Clinician II
University of Rochester
Rochester, New York

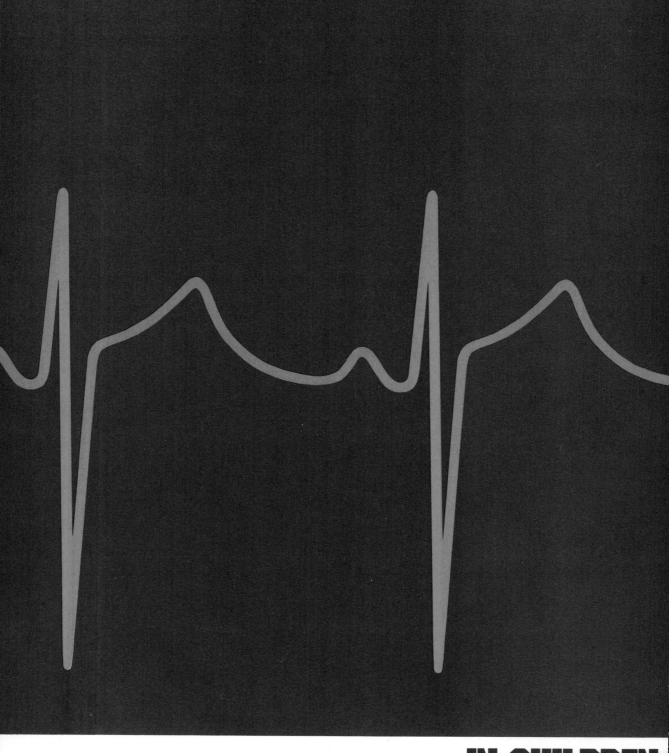

IN CHILDREN-

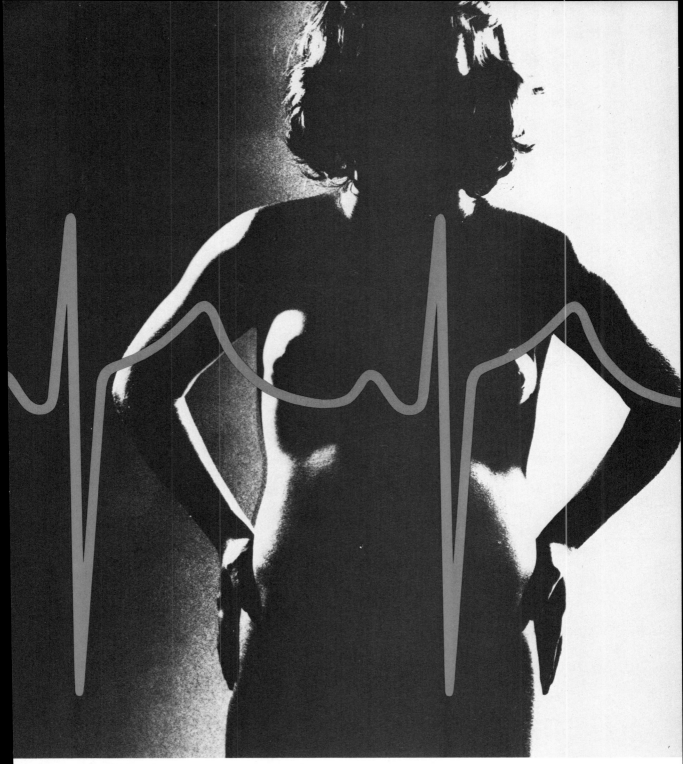

RECOGNIZE CONGENITAL ABNORMALITIES

If your patient has a water-hammer pulse accompanied by capillary pulsations of the fingernails, what cardiac abnormalities would you suspect?

What cardiac arrhythmia is most common in children?

Which common congenital anomaly causes a coarse systolic murmur at the lower left sternal border?

If your patient's receiving digoxin therapy, what electrolyte determination is it imperative to monitor prior to and during therapy?

What life-threatening complication — associated with ineffective heart-pumping action — frequently occurs in patients following cardiac surgery?

Cardiovascular Assessment
Know the norms

BY MARIE SCOTT BROWN, RN, PhD and
MARY ALEXANDER MURPHY, RN, MSN

OBVIOUSLY, MOST CHILDREN have no cardiovascular problems at all. But the unlucky ones who do are always seriously — and often fatally — ill.

Children's cardiovascular problems stem from congenital heart disease or from rheumatic fever. Congenital heart disease is the leading cause of serious illness and death in babies and newborns; rheumatic fever, the second largest cause of cardiac problems in children over age five. Even if you don't specialize in the care of children, you should know how to recognize children with these potentially fatal problems. This chapter will tell you how.

First, look at the whole child

Begin by carefully looking at the whole child. His skin tones and breathing pattern can tell you a lot. Look for the common signs of heart failure: pallor, fretfulness, inability to suckle, and uneasy breathing.

Carefully check his skin and mucous membranes, for they can tell you a lot about the health of the cardiovascular system. For example, pallor in an infant often spells severe heart problems. Look for cyanosis. It will usually appear first in the

Normal respiratory rates

AGE	RATE
Birth	30-40
1st year	26-30
2nd year	20-26
Adolescence	20

lips, nailbeds, or ear lobes. Any persistent cyanosis is a matter of serious concern. Cyanosis is often associated with polycythemia (a hematocrit over 70%, usually).

Remember that mild cyanosis may be normal in an infant, but evaluate it with care. Normal cyanosis should *not:*
- be excessive or persistent
- cover the entire body, or
- be darker in the arms than in the legs.

Report any abnormal cyanosis to a doctor, for it points to cardiovascular or respiratory difficulty. Also, look for edema of any part. It is rare in newborns, but when it occurs, it tends to appear in the eyelids.

Respiratory and other symptoms

Sometimes respiratory symptoms are just that. But they can also reflect cardiovascular problems. So, with this in mind, evaluate symptoms such as dyspnea, orthopnea, and frequent upper respiratory infections. Also think of and look for cardiovascular problems when you see certain other curious symptoms in children:
- continuous squatting and sleeping in the knee-chest position; this is almost diagnostic of a cardiac problem (usually tetralogy of Fallot)
- easy fatigability in an older child; in an infant, falling asleep immediately after taking only 2 to 2½ oz of milk
- excessively labored breathing in an infant during defecation
- anorexia, vomiting, profuse sweating
- delayed growth and development, especially in an infant (failure to thrive)
- enlarged liver
- clubbing of the fingers and toes
- enlarged heart
- pulsating neck vessels
- tachypnea without retractions.

Evaluate pulse and blood pressure

Don't overlook the importance of measuring pulse and blood pressures. They are as important to the physical examination as they are commonplace. Remember, normal values change according to the child's age. So, keep handy a list of the normal values (see page 18) to help you evaluate them correctly.

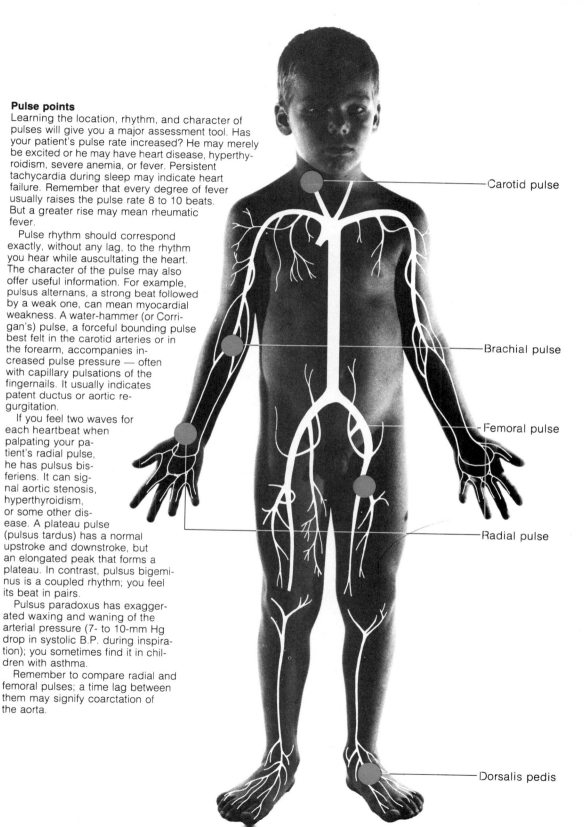

Pulse points

Learning the location, rhythm, and character of pulses will give you a major assessment tool. Has your patient's pulse rate increased? He may merely be excited or he may have heart disease, hyperthyroidism, severe anemia, or fever. Persistent tachycardia during sleep may indicate heart failure. Remember that every degree of fever usually raises the pulse rate 8 to 10 beats. But a greater rise may mean rheumatic fever.

Pulse rhythm should correspond exactly, without any lag, to the rhythm you hear while auscultating the heart. The character of the pulse may also offer useful information. For example, pulsus alternans, a strong beat followed by a weak one, can mean myocardial weakness. A water-hammer (or Corrigan's) pulse, a forceful bounding pulse best felt in the carotid arteries or in the forearm, accompanies increased pulse pressure — often with capillary pulsations of the fingernails. It usually indicates patent ductus or aortic regurgitation.

If you feel two waves for each heartbeat when palpating your patient's radial pulse, he has pulsus bisferiens. It can signal aortic stenosis, hyperthyroidism, or some other disease. A plateau pulse (pulsus tardus) has a normal upstroke and downstroke, but an elongated peak that forms a plateau. In contrast, pulsus bigeminus is a coupled rhythm; you feel its beat in pairs.

Pulsus paradoxus has exaggerated waxing and waning of the arterial pressure (7- to 10-mm Hg drop in systolic B.P. during inspiration); you sometimes find it in children with asthma.

Remember to compare radial and femoral pulses; a time lag between them may signify coarctation of the aorta.

Carotid pulse

Brachial pulse

Femoral pulse

Radial pulse

Dorsalis pedis

Know the norms

Newborn infants have rapid, fluctuating pulse rates that increase with activity or crying and decrease sharply during sleep. The irregular pulse rhythms of a newborn seem to be related to respiration. During childhood strong physical or emotional stimuli can drive the pulse rate up rapidly. You'll find a rate higher in the afternoon than in the morning and higher after meals than before. In adolescents you may find tachycardia normal, especially in girls; or, a pulse rate as slow as 40 per minute, often in athletic boys. Note, too, that during adolescence, girls' pulse rates are regularly higher than boys'. In any case, persistent tachycardia or hypertension should be investigated.

To measure arterial blood pressure accurately in small children, make sure the arm cuff covers no more than two-thirds and no less than one-half of the patient's upper arm. Blood pressure varies with the age, height, and weight of the child. You'll find many increases during adolescence: Excitement or activity can drive systolic pressure up to as much as 40 to 50 mm Hg above normal. Remember, too, that if the patient isn't quiet, you'll get a falsely high reading. Variation seems to be the rule, so know what is normal for your patient.

AVERAGE PULSE RATE AT REST				
AGE	NORMAL RANGE		AVERAGE	
Newborn	70-170		120	
1-11 months	80-160		120	
2 years	80-130		110	
4 years	80-120		100	
6 years	75-115		100	
8 years	70-110		90	
10 years	70-110		90	
	Girls	Boys	Girls	Boys
12 years	70-110	65-105	90	85
14 years	65-105	60-100	85	80
16 years	60-100	55-95	80	75
18 years	55-95	50-90	75	70

AVERAGE BLOOD PRESSURE AT REST		
AGE	GIRLS	BOYS
4 years	98/60	98/55
6 years	105/65	105/60
8 years	108/67	105/60
10 years	112/64	110/65
12 years	115/65	110/65
14 years	112/65	114/65

There are actually five sounds in a blood-pressure reading, but most clinicians cannot accurately hear them all. You should be able to hear and record at least three:

- the point at which you first hear the sounds
- the point at which they become muffled
- the point at which they disappear.

According to the American Heart Association, in children, the point of muffling should be considered the diastolic.

Next, examine the chest

To examine the chest itself, you can use inspection, palpation, percussion, and auscultation. Let's consider these in turn. Inspection of the chest is best done with the patient flat on his back, his rib cage elevated to 45 degrees. Tangential lighting is best. You can get the most accurate assessments at the end of each breath. Look for the point of maximal impulse (usually at the 5th intercostal space at the midclavicular line) and for abnormal lifts or heaves.

Also look for deformities in the shape of the chest that may alter the heart's position. Some of them, such as Marfan's syndrome (its primary lesion, dilatation of the aorta), are associated with heart problems. Others are not.

Percussion can help outline the borders of the heart but is rarely used by nurses. During *palpation* and *auscultation*, you examine five areas for any abnormal sounds, murmurs, or thrills — a sensation like holding a purring kitten.

Listen for heart sounds

A good way to auscultate is to inch your stethoscope around all five areas of the chest, first with the bell and then with the diaphragm. Do this with the child in five positions: standing, sitting straight, sitting with the chest bent forward, lying flat on the back, and lying on the left side.

Using the stethoscope, you can follow up on all the possible leads uncovered during earlier parts of the examination and look for additional ones. The first thing to check is the normalcy of heart sounds.

When listening to heart sounds, concentrate on four characteristics: rate, intensity, and rhythm of the regular sounds (see page 20), and watch for abnormal sounds — rubs, clicks, or murmurs. Evaluate the rate as you would evaluate a peripheral pulse. The apical and radial pulse should be simultaneous or at least without significant lag.

The normal heart sounds are S_1 (lub) and S_2 (dub). S_1 represents the vibration of blood in response to tricuspid and mitral valve closure. S_2 represents the vibration of blood in response to aortic and pulmonic valve closure.

Intensity of S_1 is normally greater than that of S_2 at the apex (*lub*-dub); S_2 is normally greater at the base (lub-*dub*). Increased intensity of S_1 at the base may mean recent exercise or even anemia, fever, or tachycardia. Decreased intensity of S_1 is usually more serious and can accompany an infarct. A loud S_1 with a slow heart rate (60 to 80, for instance) may mean mitral stenosis, heart block, or atrial flutter. An S_1 that constantly changes intensity, with a slow heart rate, may mean a heart block. A loud S_2 may be normal, or it may indicate coarctation or arterial hypertension.

Evaluate heart rhythm very carefully. Listen for irregularity; then decide whether it follows any pattern. If it does not, notify the doctor. The patient needs further evaluation with EKGs or a cardiac monitor. Remember, sinus arrhythmia is common in the young.

A common example of abnormal heart rhythm is *atrial*

Cuffs count

An accurate blood pressure reading depends on the proper cuff size. You should have cuffs in all the standard sizes — 2.5 inches, 5 inches, 8 inches, and 12 inches.

Since you can't easily hear the blood pressure in babies under a year old, use the flush technique. Make sure the baby is quiet, then elevate his arm or leg to drain blood from it. (This makes the arterial flow easier to hear.) Apply the blood pressure cuff, inflate it, and lower the baby's limb. As you deflate the cuff gradually, observe the point at which the limb distal to the cuff flushes with color. This is the mean systolic-diastolic pressure.

Taking thigh blood pressures can also provide helpful information. In infants, the systolic pressure in the thigh should equal that in the arm. In children older than one year, the systolic thigh pressure may be from 10 to 44 mm Hg higher than the arm pressure, but the diastolic should still be the same. If it's lower, suspect coarctation.

Don't overlook the pulse pressure — the difference between the systolic and the diastolic readings. Normally, this difference throughout childhood is about 20 to 50 mm Hg. If the pulse pressure is wide (more than 50), is it because of a low diastolic reading? If you're using the proper cuff size, then suspect a patent ductus arteriosus, aortic regurgitation, or other serious heart disease. With a high systolic reading, increased pulse pressure could be due to fever, excitement, or recent exercise. An abnormally *narrow* pulse pressure (less than 20) suggests aortic stenosis.

Sounds of the heart

- S_1: the systolic part of the cardiac cycle; the closing of the mitral and tricuspid valves makes this the "lub" of the "lub-dub"; loudest at the apex (5th ICS, midclavicular line).

- S_2: diastole; closure of the aortic and pulmonary valves at the end of systole; shorter and higher in pitch than S_1 and louder than S_1 at the base (2nd ICS); this is the "dub" of "lub-dub."

- S_3: rapid ventricular filling; occasionally heard if ventricular failure or valvular incompetency is present; a low-pitched, early diastolic sound (like the "y" in "Kentucky" where "Ken" and "tuck" represent S_1 and S_2) coming from blood rushing through the mitral and tricuspid valves, hitting empty ventricles. If caused by a left-sided dysfunction, it's best heard in the mitral area; if by a right-sided dysfunction, in the tricuspid area. This sound can be normal in a child but almost never in an adult.

- S_4: an audible atrial contraction at the very end of diastole; rapid filling into a ventricle with decreased compliance. Sounds like the "Ten" in "Tennessee" where "nes" and "see" represent S_1 and S_2; almost never normal, especially in children; more often heard in persons over 65; best heard at the apex.

- Summation gallop: all four heart sounds are present but S_3 and S_4 fuse because of a rapid heart rate (above 110 BPM); occurs in mid-diastole, best heard at the apex of the heart.

fibrillation. At first, this sounds very fast but regular. Listen more carefully, and you will realize that a few beats are being dropped. This is always abnormal. It can mean organic heart disease, rheumatic fever, thyrotoxicosis, or some other serious illness.

Common arrhythmias

The most common arrhythmia is sinus arrhythmia. The heart speeds up with inspiration and slows down with expiration. This arrhythmia does occur in normal children. To distinguish it from abnormal rhythms, you can ask an older child to hold his breath. If it is sinus arrhythmia, it should disappear. In an infant, you simply have to listen very closely to see if it fluctuates with respiration.

Bigeminy (coupled rhythm) consists of a normal beat followed by a premature contraction. Normal in some children, it may indicate organic heart disease in others. Premature beats, either atrial or ventricular, can be normal or not. Report all arrhythmias to a doctor.

Listen for unusual sounds

These come in a dizzying variety, not only S_3 and S_4, but rubs, crunches, clicks, snaps, splits, hums, and murmurs — each with meaning. S_3 is best heard at the apex with the bell of the stethoscope. It may be normal in a child, but sometimes it is really a gallop rhythm and pathological (it is always abnormal in an adult). S_3 is the diastolic (ventricular) sound that reflects rapid filling time of the ventricle. It is usually a sign of fluid overload or ventricular dysfunction. You can hear the S_4 best at the apex, too. In infants and children, it's much more rare than S_3, and is almost always abnormal. It can indicate aortic stenosis, hypertension, anemia, and hyperthyroidism. S_4 is the atrial sound at the end of diastole.

A pericardial friction rub is always abnormal. This is a scratchy, high-pitched, grating sound. It may or may not be affected by respiration. What distinguishes it from the quite similar pleural rub: The pericardial friction rub lasts only a few days; the pleural rub, much longer. Also, the pericardial friction rub extends through both systole and diastole, and you can hear it best when the patient leans forward and exhales deeply.

Hammon's sign, a mediastinal crunch, is a randomly dis-

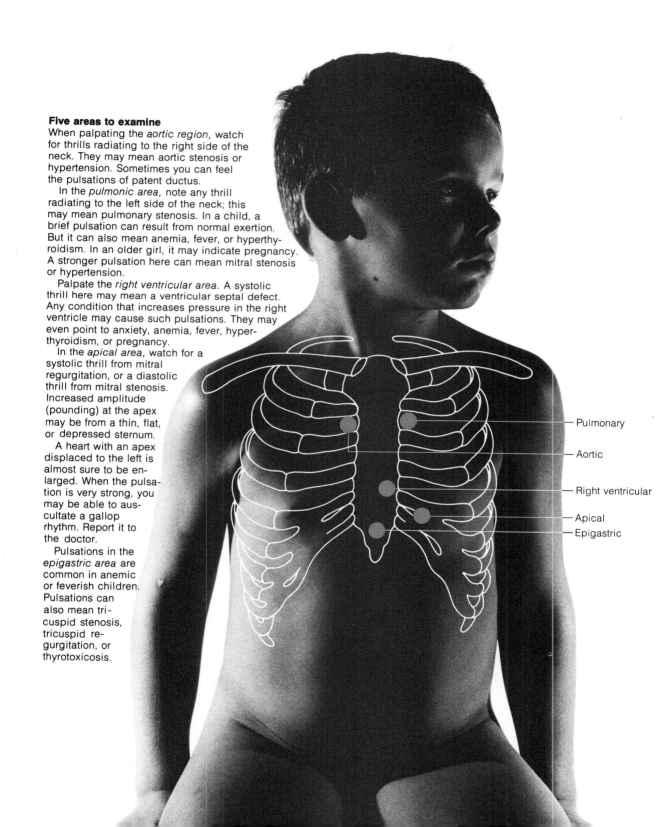

Five areas to examine

When palpating the *aortic region,* watch for thrills radiating to the right side of the neck. They may mean aortic stenosis or hypertension. Sometimes you can feel the pulsations of patent ductus.

In the *pulmonic area,* note any thrill radiating to the left side of the neck; this may mean pulmonary stenosis. In a child, a brief pulsation can result from normal exertion. But it can also mean anemia, fever, or hyperthyroidism. In an older girl, it may indicate pregnancy. A stronger pulsation here can mean mitral stenosis or hypertension.

Palpate the *right ventricular area.* A systolic thrill here may mean a ventricular septal defect. Any condition that increases pressure in the right ventricle may cause such pulsations. They may even point to anxiety, anemia, fever, hyperthyroidism, or pregnancy.

In the *apical area,* watch for a systolic thrill from mitral regurgitation, or a diastolic thrill from mitral stenosis. Increased amplitude (pounding) at the apex may be from a thin, flat, or depressed sternum.

A heart with an apex displaced to the left is almost sure to be enlarged. When the pulsation is very strong, you may be able to auscultate a gallop rhythm. Report it to the doctor.

Pulsations in the *epigastric area* are common in anemic or feverish children. Pulsations can also mean tricuspid stenosis, tricuspid regurgitation, or thyrotoxicosis.

Pulmonary

Aortic

Right ventricular

Apical

Epigastric

Listen for murmurs
Evaluate all murmurs carefully and record them as to their timing, location, radiation, intensity, pitch, and quality. Murmurs can be innocent (or functional) or organic. They can be so soft as to be almost inaudible (Grade I) or may be loud enough to be heard with the stethoscope off the chest wall (Grade VI). But only the most experienced listeners can decide whether they are innocent or not. Yet there are some clues you can keep in mind. Innocent murmurs are usually systolic, soft (Grade I or II), and transient. They are usually located at the pulmonic area, and are not transmitted. All have in common: absence of symptoms or any sign of heart disease on physical exam, EKG, or chest X-ray. They do not affect growth and development. But even these clues are not foolproof. Children with murmurs always need careful cardiac evaluation.

tributed crunching noise resulting from air in the mediastinum. It is rare but always needs attention. Report it promptly.

Clicks, splits, and hums

You may also hear clicks and ejection noises. A pulmonary ejection click is localized at the base, the anterior precordium; it lessens during inspiration or becomes louder during expiration. Pulmonary hypertension, ventricular septal defect, patent ductus, atrial septal defect, or pulmonary stenosis can cause it. An aortic ejection click occurs in early sytole at the base and at the apex: this does not change with respiration. It can be caused by aortic coarctation, aneurysm, or valve stenosis. An opening snap resembles a click but has a different quality. This sound occurs, when it does, soon after S_2 in the third or fourth left intercostal space. It results from mitral stenosis or an atrial tumor (such as myxoma).

Or you might hear one of two kinds of splits. The first is a split of the first heart sound. In some people, this sounds like a distinct, double beat over the left sternal border. It's probably normal. But if you hear a wide split or a split of the first heart sound in other areas — particularly at the apex — report it.

You may hear a venous hum, a continuous, low-pitched hum heard throughout the cycle but loudest during diastole. You can hear it best at the supraclavicular fossae, but you can also pick it up in the second-to-third intercostal space on both sides of the sternum. This hum is almost always normal, but it may mean thyrotoxicosis or anemia.

Remember these important points when assessing a child's cardiovascular system:
1. Evaluate a patient's skin and mucous membranes as well as his respirations for signs of cardiovascular irregularities.
2. Be alert for chest wall deformities that may alter the heart's position.
3. Consider heart rhythm irregularities, especially when lacking a pattern, a clue to possible cardiovascular disorders.
4. Auscultate, palpate, and percuss the chest's pulmonic, right ventricular, apical, and epigastric regions.
5. In adolescents, expect to see systolic blood pressure increase up to 40 to 50 mm Hg above normal as a result of excitement or activity.

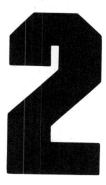

Cardiac Babies
Know six common anomalies

BY KATHY MURPHY, RN, BSN, MSN, and
KIT STAHLER-MILLER, RN, BSN, MSN

WHEN A FULL-TERM BABY with a malformed heart survives his first month of life, he is one of only about 200 such survivors his age in this country. For every such living baby, another one will have died. But at least half of those who died might have been candidates for corrective surgery — if their heart defects had been detected early enough.

Some heart defects do not show up for several years. But roughly 1% of newborns have heart defects severe enough to produce symptoms. If you work in pediatrics, or even plan to, you should know what these symptoms are and what they mean. Do you know why symptoms of congenital heart disease appear in a seemingly healthy toddler or newborn? How to assess such children accurately? Before you can answer these questions, you must understand the effects of oxygen saturation and pressure on cardiac lesions.

Oxygen saturation is simply a relative measurement (expressed as a percentage) of the amount of oxygen the hemoglobin can carry. In the normal heart, venous (right-sided) oxygen saturation is low because the tissues have extracted oxygen from the blood to meet metabolic demands; on the left side, the freshly oxygenated arterial saturation is higher because it carries deliverable oxygen to the tissues.

Pressure involves flow and resistance. Each of the four chambers in the heart has a different blood pressure (see below). Because the atria are essentially collection chambers, pressures in the atria are lower there than in the more muscular ventricles. Pressures in the left side of the heart are higher because the left ventricle pumps against high systemic resistance. The right ventricle pumps against lower pulmonary resistance and, therefore, has a lower pressure than the left ventricle. It's important to remember this. When an abnormal

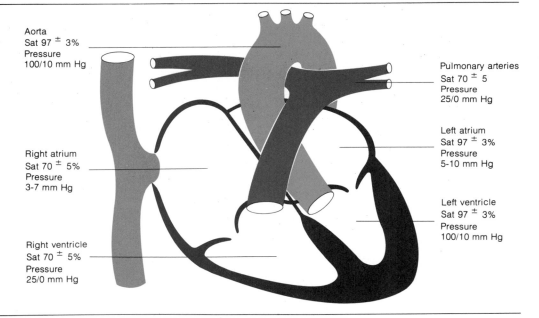

Aorta
Sat 97 $\pm$ 3%
Pressure
100/10 mm Hg

Pulmonary arteries
Sat 70 $\pm$ 5
Pressure
25/0 mm Hg

Left atrium
Sat 97 $\pm$ 3%
Pressure
5-10 mm Hg

Right atrium
Sat 70 $\pm$ 5%
Pressure
3-7 mm Hg

Left ventricle
Sat 97 $\pm$ 3%
Pressure
100/10 mm Hg

Right ventricle
Sat 70 $\pm$ 5%
Pressure
25/0 mm Hg

What's normal?
Pressures and oxygen saturation values in the heart of a newborn, as shown here, differ from those of an adult, shown on page 52.

communication exists in the heart, blood *always* flows (or shunts) from an area of higher to lower pressure.

Knowing these differences in oxygen saturation and pressure, and the structural anomalies in congenital defects, you can predict the changes in blood flow each defect can produce. With this in mind, you can plan appropriate nursing care for children with congenital heart disease. Let's review these factors in the six most common congenital defects.

Four acyanotic defects
1. *Ventricular septal defect (VSD),* the most common congen-

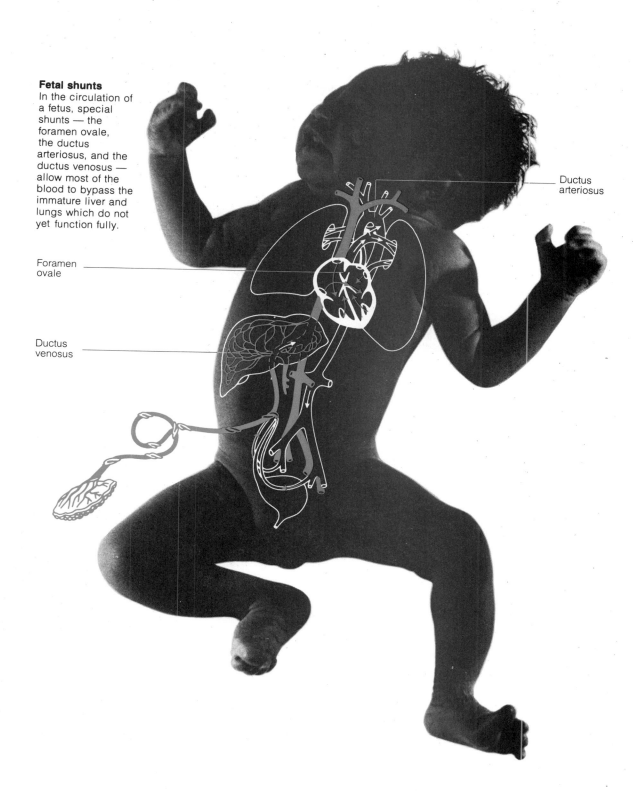

Fetal shunts
In the circulation of
a fetus, special
shunts — the
foramen ovale,
the ductus
arteriosus, and the
ductus venosus —
allow most of the
blood to bypass the
immature liver and
lungs which do not
yet function fully.

Ductus
arteriosus

Foramen
ovale

Ductus
venosus

SIX MOST COMMON ANOMALIES

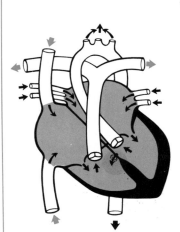

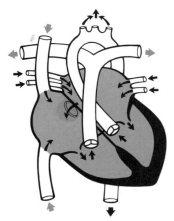

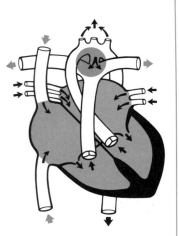

Ventricular septal defect (VSD)
One or more openings between the ventricles.

CIRCULATORY
CONSIDERATIONS
Acyanotic defect. Blood flows from area of higher to area of lower pressure. This left-to-right shunt may cause pulmonary congestion and pulmonary artery hypertension.

MURMUR
Heard in lower left sternal border; may be associated with palpable thrill. Auscultory findings depend on size of defect and amount of pulmonary vascular resistance.

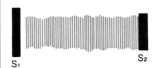

TREATMENT
Medical: CHF regimen (sedation, rest, oxygen, digoxin, sodium restriction, diuretics).
Surgical: Simple closure or patch graft with patient on cardiopulmonary bypass.

Atrial septal defect (ASD)
One or more openings between the atria. Includes ostium secundum, ostium primum, and sinus venosus.

CIRCULATORY
CONSIDERATIONS
Acyanotic defect. Left-to-right shunt may cause pulmonary congestion and pulmonary artery hypertension. Atrial arrhythmias secondary to right atrial overload and resultant interference with conduction system.

MURMUR
Systolic ejection is greatest in second and third left intercostal spaces. Fixed split S_2 on expiration heard in second, third, or fourth intercostal space.

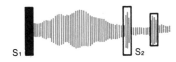

TREATMENT
Medical: Not usually necessary.
Surgical: Direct closure or patch graft with patient on cardiopulmonary bypass

Patent ductus arteriosus (PDA)
Opening between the descending aorta and bifurcation of the pulmonary artery.

CIRCULATORY
CONSIDERATIONS
Acyanotic defect. Left-to-right shunt may cause pulmonary congestion and pulmonary artery hypertension. Increased incidence in premature infants. Pulse pressure may be widened; pulses, full or bounding.

MURMUR
Continuous "machinery" murmur, greatest at upper left sternal border and under clavicle.

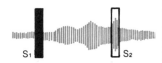

TREATMENT
Medical: CHF regimen, indomethacin for premature infants with severe respiratory distress syndrome (RDS).
Surgical: Ductal ligation in premature infants with severe RDS during neonatal period; otherwise, during toddler age.

SIX MOST COMMON ANOMALIES

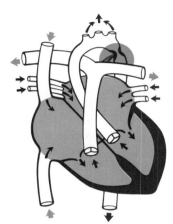

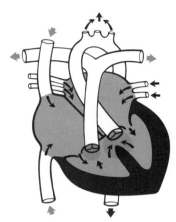

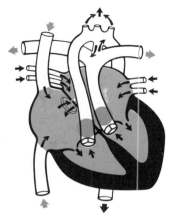

Coarctation of the aorta
Constriction of descending aorta near the ductus arteriosus.

CIRCULATORY CONSIDERATIONS
Acyanotic defect. Elevated pressures in ascending aorta and left ventricle. Insufficient mitral valve. Back pressure to lungs. Aneurysms, increased blood pressure in upper extremities, and leg cramping (may be confused with growing pains).

MURMUR
Systolic ejection click heard at base and apex of heart. Associated with systolic or continuous murmur between scapulae.

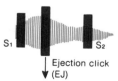

S_1

S_2

Ejection click (EJ)

TREATMENT
Medical: CHF regimen, exercise restriction.
Surgical: Resection and anastomosis, performed when patient is 6 to 12 years old.

Tetralogy of fallot
Four defects: VSD, overriding aorta, pulmonary stenosis, and right ventricular hypertrophy.

CIRCULATORY CONSIDERATIONS
Pulmonary stenosis restricts blood flow to lungs. Unoxygenated blood is shunted through the VSD. Saturated and unsaturated blood is mixed in the left ventricle and is pumped out the aorta, producing cyanosis, tet spells, clubbing, and squatting.

MURMUR
Systolic murmur and single S_2 greatest in second and third intercostal spaces at left sternal border.

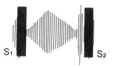

S_1

S_2

TREATMENT
Medical: CHF regimen.
Surgical: Palliative — Pott's, Blalock-Taussig, Waterston. Corrective — Close VSD and relieve pulmonary stenosis.

Transposition of great vessels
Aorta leaves right ventricle, pulmonary artery leaves left ventricle.

CIRCULATORY CONSIDERATIONS
Unoxygenated blood flows through right atrium and ventricle and out aorta to systemic circulation again. Oxygenated blood flows from lungs to left atrium and ventricle and out pulmonary artery to lungs. Sudden severe cyanosis.

MURMUR
Loud aortic closure sound at second left intercostal space. Systolic murmur with VSD.

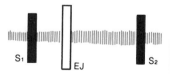

S_1

EJ

S_2

TREATMENT
Medical: Balloon septostomy, CHF regimen.
Surgical: Palliative — Blalock-Hanlen.
Corrective — Mustard, or Senning, procedure.

Cyanosis

The blue tint of cyanosis under the skin and mucous membranes comes from an abnormally high level of deoxygenated hemoglobin in capillary beds. The neonate's normal levels of hemoglobin are 16 to 22 grams/100 ml although after 1 year they will have dropped to 12 grams/100 ml. Normally 95 to 98% of this hemoglobin oxidizes in the lungs to oxyhemoglobin. With valvular or lung obstruction, extra openings in the heart chambers, or a weak pump, oxidation may be less complete. When deoxygenated levels reach 3 to 4 gram/100 ml, you may see mild cyanosis. When they climb to about 5 gram/100 ml, you'll see frank cyanosis.

Peripheral cyanosis characterizes low cardiac output. With sluggish circulation, the peripheral capillary bed constricts. In compensation, tissues extract more oxygen from the blood, leaving more deoxygenated hemoglobin.

Central cyanosis comes from inadequate oxygenation. Congenital heart defects can cause it. Pulmonary disease or obstruction leads to inadequate oxygenation at the alveolar-capillary site; this delivers less than fully saturated blood to the left atrium. The venous blood, shunted from right to left through a septal defect or a patent ductus that bypasses the lungs, may dilute the oxygen levels of the blood in the systemic circuit. In other words, abnormally deoxygenated blood is delivered to tissues which extract so much more oxygen that cyanosis becomes evident.

ital defect, allows oxygenated blood to shunt from the left to the right ventricle. Such defects may be large enough to obliterate the septum and require surgical repair. But many are small enough to close spontaneously. The opening's size and its effect on the pulmonary vasculature (the degree of congestion) determine severity of symptoms and resultant management. Tony's case was typical.

Tony is a 10-month-old infant in the cardiac clinic for progressive congestive heart failure (CHF) associated with a moderate VSD. Tony seems small but is appropriately active for his age. His mother says he's gained weight very slowly despite a good appetite. She says she fed him solid foods at 2 months because he had trouble bottle-feeding. During feedings, he needed several rest periods, became dyspneic, and sweated profusely.

While Tony sits quietly on his mother's lap, he shows no acute distress. But when he cries, he becomes dyspneic and shows mild intercostal retractions and flaring nostrils. Tony doesn't become cyanotic when he cries, but he does become very pale. If you listened to his apical heart rate, you'd find that it increased dramatically with activity, from 100 at rest to more than 160 when crying. You'd hear a coarse systolic heart murmur at his lower left sternal border and bilateral fine moist rales at the end of the inspiration. Depending on the size of the defect, you might palpate a thrill and a prominent precordial bulge. Although Tony's liver is palpable 2.5 cm below his right costal margin, he does not have edema.

Tony shows many signs common to children with right-sided congestive heart failure (see p. 26). Indeed, most children like Tony receive treatment only after developing signs of CHF. Surgical correction is usually postponed, if possible, for two reasons: some VSDs close spontaneously and, even if they do not, children tolerate heart surgery better after the age of 3.

Total correction of septal defects is done with simple closure (small-to-moderate defects) or by placement of a patch graft (large defects).

2. *Atrial septal defect (ASD)*, the second most common anomaly, is an abnormal opening between the atria. It causes changes in blood flow similar to those in VSD except for the volume of blood shunted. Because of lower pressure in the atria, ASD shunts less blood from the left to the right side.

Consequently, ASD rarely causes congestive heart failure in young children. However, the decreased systemic cardiac output from the ASD fails to deliver optimal oxygen and nutrients to the tissues. This results in impaired growth so children with ASD tend to be small for their age. Also, pulmonary overload (interstitial edema), predisposes the child to frequent respiratory infections.

Left-to-right shunts initially markedly increase pulmonary blood flow. Overcirculation of this vasculature may gradually make the vessels fibrotic and less elastic. This change produces hypertension within the pulmonary circuit and eventually reverses the intracardiac shunt from right to left.

ASD is usually corrected in late childhood to prevent permanent pulmonary vascular changes associated with pulmonary overload.

3. *Patent ductus arteriosus (PDA),* a remnant of fetal circulation (see p. 26), is an opening between the aorta and pulmonary artery. Its fetal purpose is to shunt blood away from the nonfunctional (collapsed) lungs. The ductus arteriosus normally closes spontaneously soon after birth (usually within 72 hours, but may take as long as 2 weeks). Failure to close (PDA) occurs most often in premature infants. Such infants may develop congestive heart failure because the left-to-right shunt increases blood flow to the lungs and left atrium.

Sam is a 4-month-old infant admitted for surgical ligation of a PDA. His medical records show that he was 6 weeks premature and that he required vigorous treatment (including mechanical ventilation) for respiratory distress syndrome — a disease secondary to lung immaturity.

Sam's congestive heart failure was managed with oral digitalis b.i.d. His mother says the doctors hoped digitalis would support his cardiac function until spontaneous closure of the PDA could occur. But this was a vain hope. Sam developed severe symptoms of right heart failure, similar to Tony's. If you could examine Sam, you'd see that he became dyspneic with the least exertion. You'd see tachypnea, intercostal retractions, and flaring nares; and palpate bounding axillary, femoral, and pedal pulses, and feel a thrill over his chest wall — all suggesting an A-V fistula (a runoff from the aorta to the pulmonary artery).

Sam will have surgical ligation of his PDA as soon as medical management brings his CHF under control. PDA is gener-

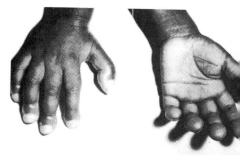

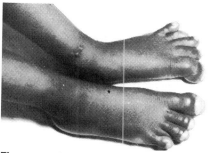

Fingers and toes
These photographs show the clubbing of the digits commonly associated with congenital heart disease, in this case with tetralogy of Fallot.

The stricken heart

A failing heart can no longer pump enough blood to meet the body's metabolic needs. When the left ventricle can't eject the volume presented to it, blood dams up behind it, engorging the pulmonary vasculature. The lungs lose compliance, and adequate gas exchange requires more effort. Recognize left heart failure by its classic signs: labored breathing with flaring nostrils, restlessness, and apprehension. Yet, in infants, tachypnea may be the only sign of impending heart failure. A sustained increase of 10 breaths a minute in a quiet, sleeping baby becomes significant. So watch for changes in respiratory rate.

In right heart failure, systemic engorgement produces distended neck veins, hepatosplenomegaly, edema of the legs (in an older child or an adult), and presacral edema. But in an infant, edema of the eyelids or face may be the first sign of heart failure (or of excessive fluid administration). Generally recumbent, infants are less likely to develop leg edema. Watch for swollen eyelids and features.

Treat heart failure with:
• rest to lighten the heart's work
• digitalis to increase the heart's power of contraction
• sodium restriction to reduce fluid retention
• diuretics to lessen edema.

ally corrected earlier than VSD because such ligation is a closed-heart procedure that doesn't require cardiopulmonary bypass and involves less risk.

4. *Coarctation of the aorta* most commonly occurs as a narrowing of the descending aorta in the area of the ductus arteriosus. It causes elevated pressures in the ascending aorta and left ventricle, which create mitral regurgitation and back pressure to the lungs. CHF may result. The increased pressure in the ascending aorta produces elevated blood pressure in the arms with possible headaches, nosebleeds, flushed cheeks, CVAs (from aneurysms, thrombosis, emboli), and lower blood pressure and cramping in the legs.

Steve, 9 years old, illustrates symptoms unique to coarctation of the aorta. Steve's school nurse first suspected his coarctation during a preschool physical examination. She noticed mild hypertension (140/100) in his arms associated with hypotension (70/50) in his legs. She palpated his pulses and found bilaterally equal and full brachial pulses, weak femorals, and bilateral absence of his pedal pulses. She referred him for cardiac evaluation, which confirmed coarctation. Since then, Steve has been healthy and has developed normally. However, because of the risk of myocardial ischemia associated with vigorous exercise, Steve has been restricted from competitive sports.

To identify children like Steve, practice good techniques for taking blood pressure in children. Always assure proper cuff size for arms and legs. Record blood pressures from all four extremities and compare the quality of brachial, radial, femoral, popliteal, and pedal pulses bilaterally. Observe for flushed cheeks, and remember to ask children about headaches or nosebleeds.

Surgical repair of coarctation is usually postponed until the child is 6 to 12 years old because the anastomosis site does not grow proportionately with the length of the aorta. Thus, postponement prevents a second surgical repair.

Two cyanotic defects

5. *Tetralogy of Fallot* includes four structural anomalies: VSD, dextroposition or overriding of the aorta, right ventricular outflow obstruction or pulmonary stenosis, and right ventricular hypertrophy. Of these four congenital cardiac defects, pulmonary stenosis and VSD are the most important

because they cause cyanosis. The pulmonary stenosis causes right ventricular hypertrophy. This causes unoxygenated blood to be shunted through the VSD into the left ventricle, where it is mixed. Thus, the ventricle pumps arterial blood with an abnormally low oxygen saturation to the systemic tissues and causes cyanosis.

Let's look at Amy, 2 years old, with confirmed tetralogy of Fallot. Her cardiac defects were confirmed by cardiac catheterization at age 3 months. Her medical management has been successful so far. But now, Amy's mother becomes very apprehensive whenever Amy shows any signs of distress. She's afraid Amy will have another "blue spell" ("tet spell") and that she might die. She says these spells are usually unpredictable, but that some happen after breakfast. During these spells, Amy becomes dyspneic and restless, her cyanosis deepens, and she gasps for breath. Usually, these spells can be relieved by placing Amy in a knee-chest position.

Recently Amy had a "blue spell" that left her unconscious but breathing for about 3 minutes. She was rushed to the emergency department, where she was found to be alert, reactive, mildly dyspneic, and cyanotic. Blood studies at that time showed mild acidosis (pH, 7.30) and polycythemia (hematocrit 65%). Amy was admitted for cardiac evaluation. If she'd had a severe "tet spell" while hospitalized, treatment would have included 100% oxygen by anesthesia mask to relieve hypoxia; morphine subcutaneously to calm her and break the dyspnea cycle; sodium bicarbonate to correct acidosis; and, possibly, propranolol (Inderal) to relieve acute dyspnea.

If you could observe Amy, you'd see obvious cyanosis even when she's resting. The cyanosis looks deepest in her lips and nail beds, but all of her skin has a dusky, bluish cast. She's slightly dyspneic. Her fingernails and toenails are clubbed, and she's small for her age.

She's small because she uses up so much of her energy (oxygen and calories) just for normal activities, such as feeding, and for coping with dyspnea, increased cardiac activity, and recurrent infection. Her dyspnea and cyanosis increase with feeding, defecation, and stress. Her "blue spells" are most likely when she's crying or has an infection.

Children like Amy know their own exercise limitations. Typically, they play and walk for a while but soon stop and squat while resting. Squatting decreases venous return and

Clues to congenital heart abnormalities

IN INFANTS
- dyspnea
- difficulty with feeding (falls asleep after taking only 2 oz of formula)
- stridor or choking spells
- pulse rate over 160
- recurrent respiratory infections
- failure to gain weight
- heart murmurs
- cyanosis
- anoxic attacks

IN CHILDREN
- dyspnea
- poor physical development
- decreased exercise tolerance
- recurrent respiratory infections
- heart murmur and thrill
- cyanosis
- squatting
- clubbing of fingers and toes
- elevated blood pressure
- absent or decreased femoral pulses
- headaches
- nosebleeds
- flushing of cheeks
- leg cramping

The goals of home care

Many parents need support to accept their child's defect immediately after his birth. Help them express their feelings so they can cope more effectively. Also, tell them what problems to expect.
• Such a child will be smaller than normal because incomplete oxygenation hinders growth.
• Such infants need more time for feedings and need to start solid food earlier, which requires less energy than sucking a bottle. Suggest small, frequent feedings that are rich in iron.
• Explain the medications their child needs as well as the purpose, dose, and side effects of each medication.
• Low-sodium diets may make the child a problem eater. Suggest appealing substitutes.
• Children with cardiac defects are vulnerable to respiratory infections and must avoid people with colds.

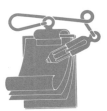

increases systemic resistance to lessen the right-to-left shunt, to improve oxygen saturation.

The increasing severity and frequency of Amy's "blue spells," coupled with polycythemia, make her a candidate for corrective surgery. Because her cyanosis results partially from a mechanical inability to perfuse her lungs, a palliative shunt may be created to increase blood flow to her lungs. Such palliative procedures (Blalock-Taussig, Waterston, and Pott's) are closed-heart methods. Total correction (with closure of VSD and relief of pulmonary stenosis) requires cardiopulmonary bypass and may be postponed until a better time.

6. *Transposition of the great vessels* occurs when the great arteries are reversed: the aorta arises from the right ventricle and the pulmonary artery arises from the left ventricle. This produces two noncommunicating circulatory systems — a condition incompatible with life. A child with this defect needs a shunt to bridge the arterial and venous systems and mix high-oxygen-saturated blood from the left heart with low-oxygen-saturated blood in the right heart. In the first few days of life, such an infant benefits from the patent ductus arteriosus. However, in a few days when this temporary pathway closes spontaneously, he quickly deteriorates. His survival depends on rapid identification of his defect and appropriate treatment.

Remember these important points when caring for infants with suspected cardiac problems:

1. Be aware that an abnormal communication in the heart causes blood to flow (or shunt) from an area of higher to an area of lower pressure.

2. Consider dyspnea and cyanosis in infants and children strong indicators of congenital heart abnormalities.

3. Recognize the signs of left heart failure: labored breathing with flaring nostrils, restlessness, and apprehension. In infants, tachypnea may be the only sign.

4. Suspect right heart failure in an infant with eyelid or facial edema.

5. Treat heart failure with rest, digitalis, sodium restriction, and diuretics.

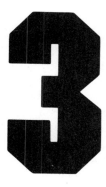

Cardiac Surgery
Know how to cope

BY KIT STAHLER-MILLER, RN, BSN, MSN, and
KATHY MURPHY, RN, BSN, MSN

DAVID, 6 YEARS OLD, is admitted for surgical closure of a large ventricular septal defect (VSD). He's one of a growing number of children hospitalized for surgical correction of congenital heart defects.

Would you feel competent to care for a child like David? To prepare him psychologically and physically for surgery? And keep track of his condition after surgery? To helpfully involve his parents? Here are some ways to do all those things well.

Your goals vary

Before surgery, your goals include preparing the child for surgery: psychologically, by telling him what to expect before, during, and after surgery without intensifying his anxiety; and, physically, while offering emotional support and reassurance. You must also prepare the child's parents so that they are able to support and reassure him throughout this terrifying crisis.

After surgery, you must know how to monitor his condition for physiologic stability, what complications to watch for and how to recognize them, and what drugs will be given and how to use them safely. And, of course, you must prepare parents to care for him during his convalescence at home. Let's look at these goals in more detail.

Expect problems at admission
Children like David are usually admitted 2 to 5 days before surgery to prepare them emotionally and physically, and to complete routine studies. Many hospitals give them and their parents a tour of the unit and information about the surgery. Even after such orientation, you'll find most children and their parents in a highly anxious state.

Parents like David's have known for a long time that surgery was inevitable for his survival. They've surely tried to prepare themselves and their child for this frightening event. Still, they can't help feeling overwhelmed by their fear of what may happen.

Parents with any unresolved guilt or inability to accept the child's defect will have much difficulty. They'll show it by being very demanding — asking many questions... looking for frequent attention for seemingly insignificant things and reasons...and even acting hostile. You need to realize this is not directed at you personally. Try to spend time with them. Allow them to express their anxiety, guilt, and frustrations. Doing so will help the child indirectly; his anxiety will, to some extent, mirror theirs.

Also remember the many sources of the child's anxiety. Many children David's age view hospitalization and painful procedures as punishment for misbehavior or bad thoughts. They are still egocentric. David's anxiety may be rooted in fear of: separation from his parents, loss of parental love, punishment, or physical harm. He may fear needles, cuts, and foreign objects on his body. He may have a heightened awareness of his body, an exaggerated concern for privacy, and may be overly modest — refuse hospital gowns, "forget" to save urine specimens, shun rectal temperatures, and deny constipation.

Older school-age children may fear abandonment, body mutilation, and death. But don't go by chronological age alone. It may be misleading. Regression is a normal and expected defense mechanism at any age: It allows the threatened person to fall back on earlier coping mechanisms. But it is frightening. The child who regresses realizes his immature inclinations, but cannot accept or control his response.

Plan teaching sessions

Before you actually begin teaching a child like David, carefully assess his developmental level, as well as his and his parents' understanding of the situation. Look for their strengths and weaknesses, as well as their ability to cope with the information you will present. Then, in uncomplicated terms, explain all aspects of the surgery to the child and his parents together. This helps the child feel more secure and allows the parents to reinforce the information later.

Watch for clues that signal the child's ability to absorb new information. If he is too anxious, he won't learn. For example, if he looks away, walks around the room, or begins to play while you're talking to him, he's had enough. When you *do* have his attention, build on what he already knows. Proceed from simple to complex explanations, discussing nonthreatening activities first. Save descriptions of threatening events (like needles) until just before they occur. Make teaching sessions short; use dolls, miniature equipment, and photographs.

Take David and his parents on a tour of the operating room (mainly by photographs) and the ICU. Introduce him to his ICU nurse. If possible, also introduce him to another child who's had similar surgery to help reassure him that he will be all right. Emphasize that not every piece of equipment that he sees will be used — just the ones you tell him about.

Give simple, honest reasons for treatments and activities. Never lie. If you lie to manipulate a child into cooperation, you'll destroy his trust and create problems. Honest explanations before painful procedures usually increase a child's tolerance of them. Be sensitive to unasked questions. Also, remember that little things can upset children the most, such as needles, not being able to have orange juice the morning of surgery, and not being able to wear underpants in the ICU.

Don't forget to tell parents how long surgery will probably last. Explain that the first 2 hours of surgery involve anesthesia, cooling, and placement of tubes. The actual corrective procedure may take less than an hour. Then, closure and re-warming will take an additional 2 hours. During surgery, try to provide brief progress reports to ease the stress of waiting.

Preoperative preparation

Physical preoperative preparation may include:
- cardiac catheterization to evaluate cardiac status

Things to tell children before cardiac surgery

- What sights and sounds (alarms and so forth) to expect in the operating room and intensive care unit.
- Monitoring equipment won't hurt.
- Catheters and monitoring equipment will be placed while he's under anesthesia and will be removed as he gets better.
- Blood on dressings and in chest tubes after surgery is normal and to be expected.
- Endotracheal intubation (call it a breathing tube) will allow periodic suctioning and it will cause him to lose his voice temporarily. Assure him that nurses will be near at all times and can read lips.
- A tube will drain urine into a bag (so he shouldn't worry about wetting the bed).
- Restraint is for protection, not punishment. Without restraint, he might pull out some of his equipment during his sleep.
- He'll be sore when he wakes up after surgery. He should tell his nurse whenever he hurts so she can give him pain medication.
- Parents will visit often, but sometimes he'll have to wait to see them.

- blood studies (CBC, BUN, and creatinine to assess renal function)
- electrolytes
- arterial blood gases (ABGs)
- coagulation profile, and type and crossmatch for donor blood
- urinalysis to evaluate his renal function
- getting an accurate weight (used to calculate fluids, electrolytes, volume replacement, and medication doses). Congestive heart failure and infections must be controlled before surgery. Some children may be given prophylactic antibiotics.

The immediate preoperative preparation varies. Some hospitals require routine antibacterial skin-cleanser baths or showers several days in advance. Others require a Betadine wash or scrub on the day before surgery. The skin shave is done from neck to knees. Tell David about the skin prep and the cleansing enema just before doing them. Afterward, explain why he can't eat or drink for a while afterwards, why wearing a hospital gown is necessary, how he'll be transported (bed or stretcher), and who'll go to the operating room with him. Explain that the preop medication will make him sleepy. Don't say it will "*put* him to sleep"; some children associate that with death.

Postoperative monitoring vital
Immediately after surgery, nursing care includes close observation and frequent reassessment of the child's physical condition. As soon as a child like David arrives from surgery, assess his cardiovascular status. His heart rate should be 70 to 100 and regular. (Heart rates for other children should be within normal limits for their age.) Monitor for arrhythmias and get a rhythm strip hourly. Arrhythmias can be expected because of surgical trauma to the conduction system, prolonged cardiopulmonary bypass, digoxin therapy, or potassium imbalance. Like some children, David could need temporary transvenous pacing.

Palpate and compare all his peripheral pulses to assess cardiac function. Dangerous signs of poor cardiac output: cool, clammy skin; mottling; poor capillary refill; and urine output less than 1 ml/kg/hour.

After cardiac surgery, David had intracardiac catheters, (CVP, PAP/wedge) connected to an oscilloscope to measure

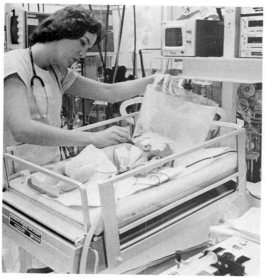

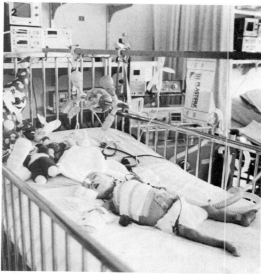

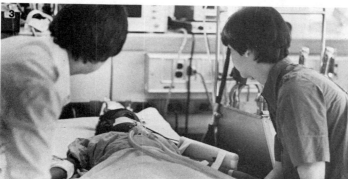

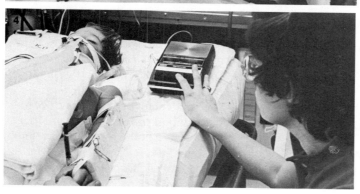

Aftermath of cardiac surgery

Recovering from cardiac surgery is an enormous job. A child can easily become overwhelmed by the strange environment and frightening equipment. Here are some things you can do to make his course easier.

First, cope with your own anxiety so you don't pass it along to your patient. Know what to expect so you're prepared for any situation.

Second, to make the child feel more comfortable and less lost, place toys and other familiar objects from home within his sight.

Third, talk to your patient when you give physical care. Reassure him with a touch or by the tone of your voice that everything will be OK.

Fourth, hospitalized children can be comforted by hearing the voices of family and friends on a cassette tape recorder.

Show that you care

Even the best prepared child will feel lost and frightened in a hospital situation. You can foster some sense of security by continually reassuring him by words and actions that you will try to meet his needs.

For example, assure his comfort by controlling pain. Give pain medication half an hour before painful procedures and whenever he seems restless or cannot sleep. Relieving pain helps prevent feelings of anger and loss of control and encourages cooperation.

Remember that immobility, multiple tubes, and the imposition of treatments can cause feelings of helplessness. So return as much control as possible. Offer simple choices like asking your patient when he wants to bathe or sit in a chair. This allows him to cope in his own way with unpleasant situations.

Above all, involve parents in nursing care whenever possible. This helps fill parental needs and fosters security for them and the child.

blood pressures within his various heart chambers. Report all variations from normal limits. Watch for an increased CVP (central venous pressure) associated with decreased intra-arterial pressure, or increased pulmonary artery pressure and other signs of left-sided heart failure (frothy endotracheal secretions, dyspnea, cough, and pulmonary rales). Heart failure may be secondary to volume overload and a damaged conduction system.

Another postop problem to worry about: cardiac tamponade. It occurs when the heart gets compressed in the mediastinal space by clotted or unclotted blood and can't function effectively as a pump. *It's an extreme emergency* and requires immediate thoracentesis or thoracotomy. Watch for its signs: sudden increase or decrease in the chest tube drainage accompanied by decreased blood pressure, narrowed pulse pressure, increased CVP, engorged neck veins, and pulsus paradoxus (a marked decrease in pulse amplitude with inspiration).

If David was receiving digoxin, the doctor may order it resumed postoperatively. *Caution:* Because of the hazards of digoxin in persons with hypokalemia, always get *a serum potassium before beginning digoxin treatment.* Thereafter, check the serum potassium level every 2 to 3 days, or as ordered.

Respiratory care vital

Note whether David's respirations are spontaneous or respirator-dependent. They should be regular at a rate of 20 to 22 per minute. Watch for signs of respiratory distress — tachypnea, dyspnea, retractions, flaring nares, grunting, prolonged expiration, duskiness, or cyanosis. Look for bilateral equal expansion of his chest wall. Auscultate breath sounds for bilateral equality of aeration, absence of aeration in any area(s), or accessory sounds such as rales, rhonchi, or rubs (over the anterior chest). Monitor arterial blood gases to assess ability to oxygenate and remove CO_2.

Pneumothorax is a potential complication of both cardiac surgery and mechanical ventilation. A tension pneumothorax is a collection of air under pressure in the pleural space which compromises lung expansion. Suspect it when you find an absence of breath sounds accompanied by a gradual or sudden increase in dyspnea. Prompt insertion of a chest tube can reestablish the negative intrapleural pressure and help to relieve distress.

At most hospitals, a portable chest X-ray is used immediately after surgery and then daily to view lung reexpansion and heart size. Two chest tubes (one, a mediastinal tube) are generally in place. These tubes are usually connected to a portable drainage system, which is connected to wall suction. These tubes need frequent and careful milking or stripping to prevent clot formation. Record the amount, color, and consistency of the drainage hourly. Total these amounts at the end of your shift and record them in your notes. Tape the same information on the Pleur-evac with your initials, the time, and the date.

Watch for complications

Guard against hypovolemia, a frequent complication due to inadequate postoperative blood replacement. To evaluate the adequacy of blood and fluid replacement, monitor intracardiac pressures, the amount of chest tube drainage, and urine output. Hypovolemia can lead to poor renal perfusion and renal shutdown, so maintain adequate urine output. Body weight is the final index of fluid balance, so weigh the child at the same time each day, on a bedside scale.

Check serum electrolytes. Initially, you'll need to check David's electrolytes at least every 4 hours because rapid shifts can occur. You may see hyponatremia (dilutional), which the doctor will treat with diuretics and decreased water intake. However, you must watch most zealously for electrolyte shifts that may cause arrhythmias. Hypokalemia may cause dizziness, hypotension, EKG changes, and cardiac arrest. And hypokalemia and hypocalcemia intensify the patient's sensitivity to digoxin (Lanoxin).

Monitor hematologic studies. Hemoglobin and hematocrit are indexes of hydration as well as other functions. Clotting studies (prothrombin time and partial thromboplastin time) are ordered to check reversal of heparinization by protamine during surgery. The platelet count tells the degree of platelet destruction by the membrane oxygenator. Blood urea nitrogen (BUN) and creatinine levels provide a renal function index.

Assess neurologic status. Complications of the membrane oxygenator are thrombi, emboli, and cerebral anoxic damage. All can impair neurologic function. Repeatedly evaluate pupil equality and reaction to light, equal movement and sensation in extremities, level of consciousness, and response to commands.

Convalescence after ICU
A patient like David will probably need treatment in the ICU for at least 2 days. As he improves, his supportive equipment will be removed. Then, he and his parents may need reassurance that intensive monitoring and observation are no longer necessary and that he can be cared for just as well on the medical-surgical unit.

Children like David need postoperative care for about another week before they can be discharged. Nursing care during this early convalescence includes observation for, and prevention of, infection in the incisional areas; chest hygiene (postural drainage and percussion to maintain pulmonary functions and prevent respiratory infections); continued assessment of breath sounds; and regular cardiovascular assessments.

Maintaining fluid and electrolyte balance remains important during early convalescence. The child may need fluid restriction and a low-sodium diet to decrease the work load on the healing heart muscle. Be sure to explain the reason for this and other restrictions to the parents during your discharge teaching.

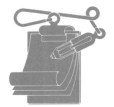

Remember these important points when preparing a child for cardiac surgery:
1. Clearly explain to your patient and his parents what to expect before, during, and after surgery. Offer emotional support and reassurance.
2. Allow the child and his parents to express feelings of anxiety and guilt.
3. Expect preoperative preparations to include cardiac catheterization, serum electrolyte and ABG studies, blood coagulation profile and type and cross match, urinalysis, and an accurate weight reading.
4. Gear teaching sessions to the child's developmental level and to his ability to absorb new information.
5. After surgery, closely monitor and frequently reassess your patient for signs of complications, such as cardiac arrhythmias, increased CVP, sudden increase or decrease in chest tube drainage, serum electrolyte shifts, hematologic disturbances, and neurologic impairments.

SKILLCHECK

1. Sally, 6 months old, is admitted to your pediatric unit for cardiac evaluation. Her skin looks dusky when she cries. When you take her pulse, you feel a forceful bounding quality over both the radial and femoral pulses. What diagnosis do you suspect?

2. When you take Sally's blood pressure, you hear pulse sounds begin, become muffled, and then disappear. Which point is the diastolic blood pressure?

3. Bill, 9 months old, is hospitalized for upper respiratory infection. When you listen to his heart, you notice that S_1 and S_2 are followed by a distinct low-pitched sound that you hear best at the apex. What is it and what should you do about it?

4. Tommy is 9 years old. When you take his apical pulse, you notice that his heart rate speeds up with inspiration and slows down with expiration. What does this mean?

5. Which of the following is *not* a symptom of cardiac disease in a 3-month-old infant: falling asleep after taking 2 oz. of milk; clubbing of fingers and toes; S_3 on auscultation; or failure to gain weight?

6. In children, a narrow pulse pressure (less than 20 mm Hg) suggests which of the following: patent ductus arteriosus; aortic stenosis; tetralogy of Fallot; or aortic regurgitation?

7. In children born with tetralogy of Fallot, a common compensation by the body for low arterial oxygen saturation is... fatigue, high blood pressure, right ventricular hypertrophy, or polycythemia?

8. Children with cardiac defects are often hospitalized with respiratory infections. Why are they susceptible to these infections? Is the mechanism the same in acyanotic and cyanotic disorders?

9. Following cardiac surgery, cool and clammy skin, poor capillary refill, and low urine output are ominous signs of: decreased renal function, cardiac tamponade, hypertensive crisis, or low cardiac output?

10. Paul has just returned from surgery where his ventricular septal defect was repaired. You notice that he is having 6 to 10 PVCs (premature ventricular contractions) per minute. What does this mean and what should you do?

(Answers on page 171)

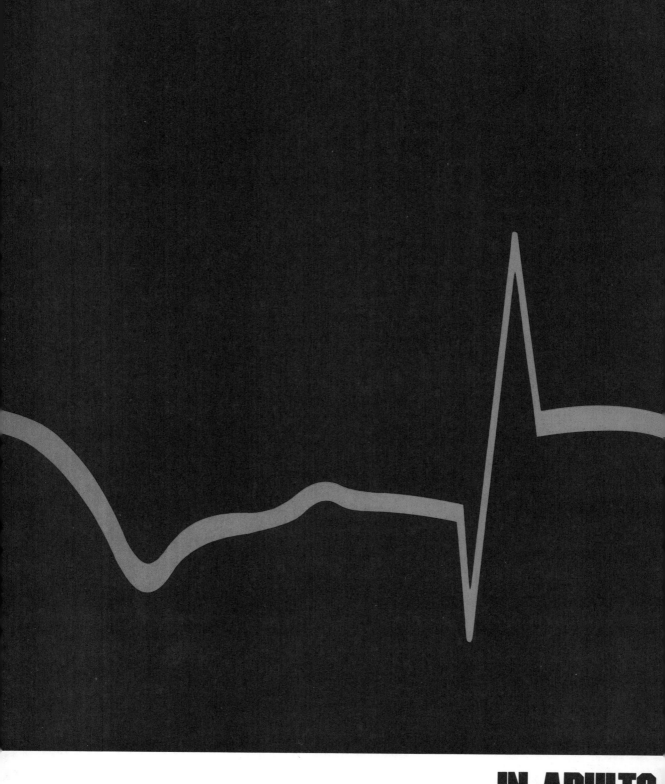

IN ADULTS:

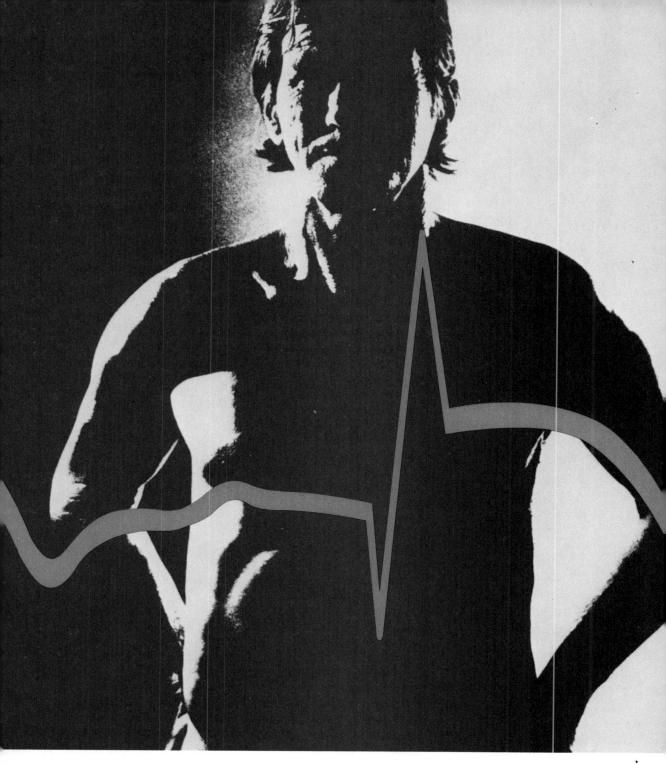

DEAL WITH ACQUIRED DISEASE

How does a beta blocker control
hypertension?

If your patient has chest pain, what questions
should you ask to rule out angina?

What complication frequently occurs in a
patient with a myocardial infarction?

What are your nursing responsibilities when
caring for a patient in the interstitial stage
of pulmonary edema?

If you're weaning a patient from an
intraaortic balloon pump, what signs and
symptoms would tell you to stop
the weaning procedure?

If your patient with heart failure,
arrhythmias, and embolic phenomena
has an enlarged heart, gallop rhythms,
and valvular insufficiency, what type of
cardiomyopathy should you suspect?

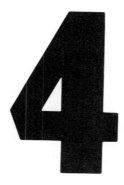

Assessment
Review of vital skills

BY CHRISTINE SUE BREU, RN, BSN, MN

CAREFUL ASSESSMENT IS ONE of your most vital contributions to the care of patients with cardiovascular problems. During the initial assessment, it's your assignment to collect all pertinent information about the patient's present condition and his medical history. This careful evaluation helps pinpoint the source of the problems, sets a reliable baseline against which to measure the effectiveness of treatment, and helps you to plan comprehensive care.

Don't overlook the history
In haste to identify the patient's problem, you may be tempted to overlook the medical history. Yet the subjective information the patient himself can give you may be crucial. Always remember to define the patient's chief complaint — the patient's description in his own words of what caused him to seek medical help. You might ask, ''What brought you to the hospital (or doctor's office)?'' Find out how long the patient's had the problem, how it's affected his life-style, the details surrounding its onset, and any causative factors. Be sure to elicit a full description of the symptoms, including location, radiation, intensity, and duration; any associated symptoms, and the

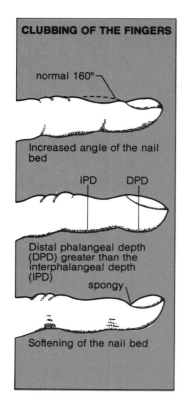

CLUBBING OF THE FINGERS

normal 160°

Increased angle of the nail bed

IPD   DPD

Distal phalangeal depth (DPD) greater than the interphalangeal depth (IPD)

spongy

Softening of the nail bed

effect of any treatment or medications.

Next, proceed with inspection, auscultation, palpation, and percussion.

Begin with inspection

Look at the patient. Does he seem anxious or calm, tired or energetic? Does he seem to be in any distress?

Look for and ask about skin changes. Remember that insufficient circulation can produce dry, brittle hair; dry, shining skin; and thickened nails (especially on the toes). Check for skin color:

• *Cyanosis* may indicate a congenital heart anomaly, congestive heart failure, or various pulmonary diseases. But keep in mind the difference between peripheral and central cyanosis. Peripheral cyanosis is on the fingertips and lips. It's not necessarily a sign of disease; you can see it in patients who are cold or anxious. Central cyanosis causes blue coloration in the mouth and on the lips, as well as in the nail beds. It usually indicates a major oxygenation deficiency that accompanies heart and lung diseases.

• *Jaundice* occurs in late congestive heart failure. It results from an increased bilirubin level. It's easiest to see in the sclerae under natural light.

• *Generalized pallor* can result from decreased levels of oxygenated hemoglobin (as in anemia). Pallor is often hard to evaluate because of individual variations in skin coloring. It's usually easiest to see in the conjunctivae, mouth, and nails.

Look for clubbing of the nails. It's common in patients with lung cancer, chronic obstructive lung disease, and congenital cardiovascular disease. To distinguish between normal, familial roundness of the nails and clubbing, examine the angle between the nail bed and the finger. An angle greater than 160 degrees suggests clubbing (see insert).

Another sign of clubbing is an increase in the diameter of the fingertip that makes the distal phalangeal depth (DPD) greater than the interphalangeal depth (IPD). Also, watch for softening of the nail bed — a sign of chronic hypoxia.

Pay particular attention to venous distention or abnormal pulsation in the neck. These conditions can indicate right-sided heart failure, right-sided valvular disease, or cardiac tamponade. When assessing distention, use the internal jugular vein. Your reference point is the angle at which the manubrium fuses with the sternun (see insert). Record the estimated jugular venous distention as normal, increased, or markedly increased, along with the level of the head of the bed when you made the observation.

Proceed with inspection of the anterior chest in a systematic way. Concentrate on five areas: the aortic area, the second intercostal space to the right of the sternum; the pulmonic area, the second intercostal space to the left of the sternum; the right ventricular area, the lower half of the left sternal border; the apical area, the fifth intercostal space along the midclavicular line; and the epigastric area, near the xiphoid process. Carefully inspect each area for pulsations. Later you'll correlate these observations with other findings.

Palpation next

Feel the skin for temperature and moisture. Evaluate skin turgor by lifting a fold of the skin to see how promptly it returns to normal. Sluggish return to normal could mean dehydration. Also check for edema, especially in the legs, sacrum, and other dependent areas. Press swollen areas with your fingers to see if indentions result (pitting edema).

Carefully assess all peripheral pulses. Include the carotids, brachials, radials, femorals, popliteals, dorsalis pedis, and posterior tibials. Note their rate, quality, and equality. They should be bilaterally equal. Rate the pulses on a scale of 0 to 4 +: 0, absent; 1 +, barely palpable; 2 +, normal or average; 3 +, full; and 4 +, full, bounding, and often visible. (See insert, page 49, for the way they should test.)

When assessing arterial pulses, you may find pulsus alternans. This is a variation in pulse in which weak impulses alternate with strong impulses. If you suspect pulsus alternans, apply a blood pressure cuff and elevate the pressure above the systolic level. Then gradually lower the pressure. At first you'll hear only the stronger beats. Then the pulse rate will double as the cuff pressure is lowered, and you'll hear weaker beats, too. Pulsus alternans can indicate ventricular failure.

Another abnormal sign is a paradoxical pulse. Normally, the systolic blood pressure falls slightly (4 to 8 mm Hg) during inspiration. With paradoxical pulse, the fall is greater than 10 mm Hg. To detect it, apply a blood pressure cuff and raise the pressure to the systolic level so you hear beats on expira-

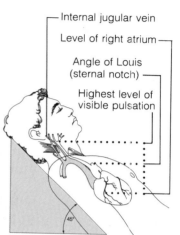

- Internal jugular vein

Level of right atrium

Angle of Louis (sternal notch)

Highest level of visible pulsation

Estimating venous pressure
This illustration shows how to measure venous pressure indirectly. Place the patient at a 45° angle. Observe the internal jugular vein to determine the highest level of visible pulsation. (Although you can use the external or the internal jugular vein, the internal jugular is the more reliable indicator of venous pressure.)

Next, locate the angle of Louis, or sternal notch. To do so, palpate the clavicles where they join the sternum (the suprasternal notch). Place your first two fingers on the suprasternal notch. Then, without lifting them from the skin, slide them down the sternum until you feel a bony protuberance—the angle of Louis.

To estimate venous pressure, measure the vertical distance between the highest level of visible pulsation and the angle of Louis. Normally, this vertical distance is less than 3 cm. Add 5 cm to this figure to estimate the total distance between the highest level of pulsation and the right atrium. If your total exceeds 10 cm, consider venous pressure elevated and suspect right heart failure.

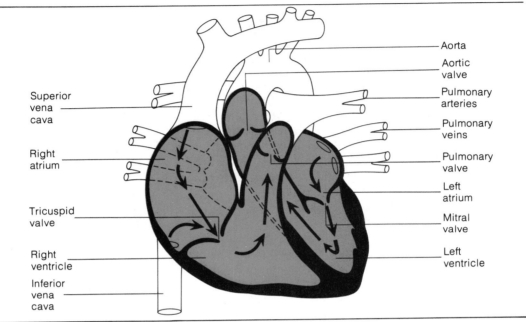

Life's blood
This illustration shows the normal circulation of blood through the heart.

tion. Slowly deflate the cuff to the point where you hear impulses during both inspiration and expiration. The difference between the first reading and the second is the paradoxical pulse. It points to possible constrictive pericarditis, cardiac tamponade, or pulmonary emphysema.

Palpate the chest in the same systematic way you used for inspection. In the same areas (aortic, pulmonic, right ventricular, apical, and epigastric), carefully palpate for pulsations or thrills (cat-purring vibrations). Use the ball of the hand to feel thrills, the finger pads to feel pulsations. If you find either, you'll have to correlate it with the heart sounds or with the carotid pulse.

In the apical area, pay special attention to the apical impulse. It's normally found in the fifth intercostal space at the left midclavicular line. This is usually called the point of maximal impulse (PMI). It correlates with ventricular systole and gives valuable information about abnormalities of the left ventricle. The PMI is usually only 2 cm in diameter, begins with the first heart sound, and lasts only to midsystole. If it's larger or more lateral than normal, it could indicate left-sided valvular disease, coronary artery disease, or hypertension. If it's sustained and forceful, it could indicate left ventricular hypertrophy. You may detect left ventricular gallops in this same area. In patients with right ventricular hypertrophy, you will feel a lift in the left parasternal area during systole.

Percussion

Percussion will help you determine heart size. But remember, this procedure is rarely included in a routine cardiac examination.

Percussion techniques used in examining the heart are the same as those for examining the lungs. With the patient lying down, begin to percuss his chest at the anterior axillary line. Start at the fifth intercostal space and move to the fourth, if necessary; percuss toward the sternum until you hear dullness. When you hear the change in the note, you have found the left border of cardiac dullness (LBCD). In the average adult male this is near the point of maximal impulse, usually 10 to 12 cm from the midsternal line and always within the midclavicular line (MCL). If the LBCD is greater than 12 cm from midsternum and outside the MCL, the heart may be enlarged. Only in a highly trained athlete can this be considered a normal finding.

If you have noticed anything abnormal so far, set out to confirm it through auscultation.

Auscultation

The key to successful auscultation is focusing on one sound at a time. Listen for S_1 and S_2 and then systole and diastole. Before you can do this you must have a thorough grasp of the hemodynamic events that occur in the cardiac cycle. Review these events repeatedly until you know them well enough to identify each element of the cardiac cycle... when each valve opens and closes... systole and diastole.

For accurate auscultation, the stethoscope must be equipped with both a diaphragm (to hear higher-pitched sounds) and a bell (to hear lower-pitched sounds). Remember, the bell is effective only when placed very lightly on the chest wall.

Proceed with auscultation in a systematic and orderly fashion. Each heart valve and its related sounds are reflected to a specific area of the chest wall. You hear the aortic valve sounds best in the second intercostal space to the right of the sternum; pulmonic sounds, in the second intercostal space to

Assessing peripheral pulses
Assess peripheral pulses bilaterally, noting their rate, quality, and equality. Here's how they should test:

	Right	Left
Temporal	2+	2+
Carotid	3+	3+
Brachial	2+	2+
Femoral	2+	2+
Popliteal	2+	2+
Posterior tibial	2+	2+
Dorsalis pedis	2+	2+

the left of the sternum; tricuspid sounds, in the fifth intercostal space near the left sternal border; and mitral sounds, in the fifth intercostal space near the midclavicular line. To be sure your auscultation is thorough, start at the aortic area and inch your way to each of the other valvular areas. Perform this procedure once with the diaphragm and then once using the bell.

S_1 — The first heart sound

At the beginning of ventricular systole, after the atria have been stimulated to contract, pressure rises in the ventricles to the point where it becomes higher than atrial pressure. At this point, the atrioventricular valves — the tricuspid on the right side and the mitral on the left side — are forced closed. As this occurs, the first heart sound (S_1) is transmitted to the chest wall. Since it's associated with mitral and tricuspid valve closure, this sound is normally loudest at the apex of the heart (around the fifth intercostal space at the left midclavicular line). Normally, the mitral valve closes slightly before the tricuspid valve, but they are so close together that only one sound is heard. If for some reason the valve closure is separated, you can hear a splitting of S_1. When listening to S_1, listen carefully for intensity, consistency, and splitting.

S_2 — The second heart sound

As the cardiac cycle continues, after the atrioventricular valves close (S_1), the ventricle goes into the ejection phase of systole. This increased pressure forces open the semilunar valves — the pulmonic valve on the right side and the aortic valve on the left side. As systole ends and the ventricle starts to relax, there's a slight backflow of blood in the pulmonary artery and in the aorta. This backflow causes the pulmonic valve and the aortic valve to close. The sound transmitted to the chest wall at this time is the second heart sound (S_2). Since this sound is associated with pulmonic and aortic valve closure, S_2 is loudest at the base of the heart (the second intercostal space). Normally, the aortic valve closes before the pulmonic valve but they're so close together that only one sound is heard. If the valve closures separate, you can hear a splitting of S_2.

Listen to S_2 for intensity, consistency, and splitting. Since S_1 occurs at the beginning of systole and S_2 at the end of systole, the pause between S_1 and S_2 contains systolic sounds;

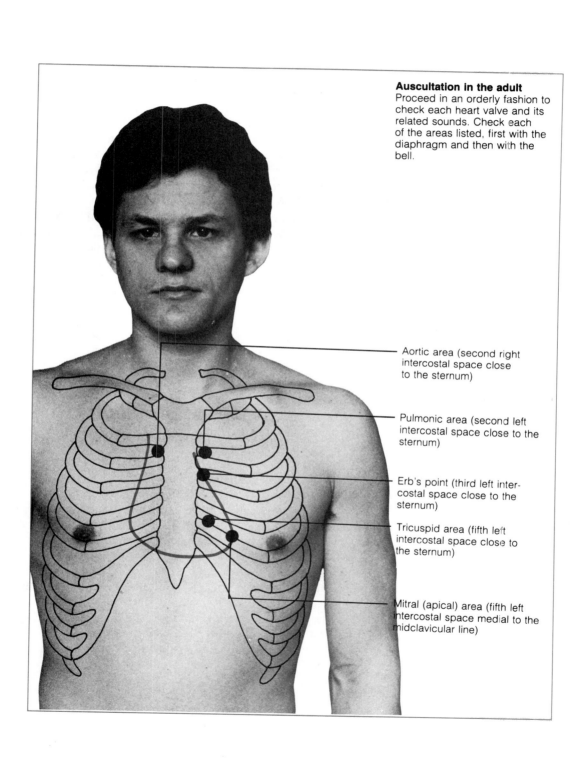

Auscultation in the adult
Proceed in an orderly fashion to check each heart valve and its related sounds. Check each of the areas listed, first with the diaphragm and then with the bell.

Aortic area (second right intercostal space close to the sternum)

Pulmonic area (second left intercostal space close to the sternum)

Erb's point (third left intercostal space close to the sternum)

Tricuspid area (fifth left intercostal space close to the sternum)

Mitral (apical) area (fifth left intercostal space medial to the midclavicular line)

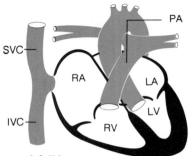

A full heart
The normal blood pressures and oxygen saturation levels in an adult heart are as follows:

SUPERIOR VENA CAVA (SVC)
Pressure — 2 to 14 mm Hg
(maximum mean range)
0 to 8 mm Hg
(minimum mean range)
Oxygen — 70% to 87%

INFERIOR VENA CAVA (IVC)
Pressure — same as SVC
Oxygen — 77% to 85%

RIGHT ATRIUM (RA)
Pressure — $\dfrac{2\ to\ 14}{-2\ to\ +6}$ mm Hg
Oxygen — 74% to 86%

RIGHT VENTRICLE (RV)
Pressure — $\dfrac{15\ to\ 28}{0\ to\ 8}$ mm Hg
Oxygen — 71% to 87%

PULMONARY ARTERY (PA)
Pressure — $\dfrac{15\ to\ 28}{5\ to\ 16}$ mm Hg
Pulmonary wedge (PW)
Pressure — 6 to 15 mm Hg
(mean range)
Oxygen — 73% to 83%

LEFT ATRIUM (LA)
Pressure — $\dfrac{6\ to\ 20}{-2\ to\ +9}$ mm Hg
Oxygen — 94% to 100%

LEFT VENTRICLE (LV)
Pressure — $\dfrac{90\ to\ 140}{4\ to\ 12}$ mm Hg
Oxygen — 94% to 100%

the pause between S_2 and the next S_1 contains diastolic sounds.

S_3 — The third heart sound

The next event in the cardiac cycle is the resting phase of the ventricles (diastole). At the beginning of diastole, the pressure in the atria exceeds the pressure in the ventricles and causes the mitral and tricuspid valves to open. This allows a very rapid filling phase of the ventricles as the blood in the atria rushes into the ventricles. This sets up low-frequency vibrations that are normally inaudible, but you may detect them in some normal children and young adults, in patients with valvular regurgitation, or in those with ventricular failure. These low-frequency sounds constitute the third heart sound, or S_3. It's also called a diastolic filling sound or a ventricular gallop. It's heard best with the bell of the stethoscope when the patient lies in the left lateral position.

When S_3 results from left ventricular failure or aortic or mitral valvular regurgitation, it's heard best over the mitral area. If it results from right ventricular failure or right valvular regurgitation, it's heard best in the tricuspid area. Since an S_3 occurs at the beginning of diastole and a split S_2 occurs at the end of systole, you must listen carefully at different places to distinguish between these two sounds.

S_4 — The fourth heart sound

Ventricular filling continues throughout diastole and ends with atrial contraction. This is a slow filling phase of the ventricle that creates low-frequency sounds which, when audible, are the fourth heart sound, or S_4. An S_4 is often found in patients with a decreased ventricular compliance (in hypertension, semilunar valvular stenosis, coronary artery disease, or an acute myocardial infarction). It's often heard in older patients, especially those over 65. It's also called a diastolic filling sound or an atrial gallop sound. Since it, too, is a low-frequency sound, listen for it with the bell of the stethoscope (with the patient lying in the left lateral position).

If S_4 results from left-sided dysfunction, you can hear it best in the mitral area; if from right-sided dysfunction, you can hear it best in the tricuspid area.

Since an S_4 occurs at the end of diastole and a split S_1 occurs at the beginning of systole, you must listen carefully to distin-

HOW VARIOUS KINDS OF CARDIAC PAIN DIFFER				
	ONSET AND DURATION	LOCATION AND RADIATION	QUALITY AND INTENSITY	SIGNS AND SYMPTOMS	PRECIPITATING FACTORS
MYOCARDIAL INFARCTION	Sudden onset; pain ½ to 2 hours; residual soreness 1 to 3 days	Substernal, midline, or anterior chest pain; radiation to jaws, neck, back, shoulders, or one or both arms	Severe pressure; deep sensation — "crushing," "squeezing," "indigestion"	Apprehension, nausea, dyspnea, diaphoresis, increased blood pressure, gallop rhythm	Occurrence at rest or with exertion — physical or emotional
ANGINA	Gradual or sudden onset; pain usually lasts less than 15 minutes	Substernal or anterior chest pain, not sharply localized; radiation to back, neck, arms, jaw, even upper abdomen or fingers	Mild-to-moderate pressure, uniform pattern of attacks; deep sensation, tightness — "squeezing"	Dyspnea, diaphoresis, nausea, desire to void, belching, apprehension	Exertion, stress, eating, micturition, or defecation; cold or hot, humid weather
PERICARDITIS	Sudden onset; continuous pain lasting for days; residual soreness	Substernal pain to left of midline; radiation to back or subclavicular area	Mild ache to severe pain, deep or superficial — "stabbing," "knife-like"	Precordial friction rub; increased pain with movement, inspiration, laughing, coughing, left side position; decreased pain with sitting or leaning forward	Bacterial, fungal, or viral infection; postcardiac injury, such as myocardial infarction, trauma, or surgery; no relation to effort

guish these sounds, their location, pitch, timing, and duration.

Quadruple rhythm

Occasionally, you can hear both S_3 and S_4 along with S_1 and S_2. This is called a quadruple rhythm. If this rhythm occurs in a patient whose pulse rate is faster than 110 beats per minute, the third and fourth heart sounds fuse to make one middiastolic sound. This is called a summation gallop.

Murmurs

Murmurs are sounds produced by abnormal turbulence. This turbulence can be caused by valvular or septal wall pathology or by anemia. Murmurs are classified according to timing, intensity, location, pitch, quality, and radiation.

When timing a murmur, you must establish if it occurs during diastole or during systole. Remember, if you hear a murmur between S_1 and S_2, it's a systolic murmur; between S_2 and the next S_1, it's a diastolic murmur. Fine timing is deciding exactly where in systole or in diastole the murmur occurs — for example, middiastole or late systole.

Grade the intensity of the murmur from I to VI. Grade I is very faint; II is soft and low; III is prominent but not palpable; IV is prominent and palpable (you can feel a thrill); V can be heard with the stethoscope held 1″ from the chest wall; and Grade VI is audible without a stethoscope.

Murmurs that occur during systole (because of left-sided pathology) are the murmurs of aortic stenosis and mitral regurgitation. Those that occur during systole (because of right-sided pathology) are the murmurs of pulmonic stenosis and tricuspid regurgitation. Murmurs that occur during diastole (when the left ventricle is filling) are the murmurs of mitral stenosis and aortic regurgitation. Murmurs that occur during diastole (when the right ventricle is filling) are the murmurs of tricuspid stenosis and pulmonic regurgitation.

Pericardial friction rub

In patients who have pericarditis, you may hear a pericardial friction rub. This is a high-pitched, scratchy sound that seems close to the listener's ear. It can have three components: atrial systole, ventricular systole, and ventricular diastole. You can hear a pericardial friction rub best with the diaphragm of the stethoscope when the patient leans forward. The sound comes and goes without any discernible pattern. It's usually located around the fourth or fifth intercostal space from the sternal border to the apex.

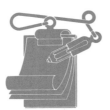

Remember these important points when assessing an adult's cardiovascular system:
1. Determine how your patient's problem has affected his life-style, so you can plan patient teaching and foster appropriate coping skills.
2. Suspect a cardiovascular problem if you see these skin color changes: cyanosis, jaundice, or generalized pallor.
3. Be aware that a PMI larger than 1 or 2 cm in diameter may indicate left-sided valvular disease, coronary artery disease, or hypertension.
4. Know that heart sounds reflect the noise made by blood rerouting as a result of valve closures.
5. Differentiate murmurs by timing, quality, location, pitch, and radiation.

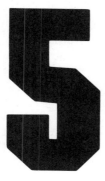

Diagnostic Tests
Invasive and noninvasive

BY ARLENE B. STRONG, RN, MN

DEFINING A PATIENT'S CARDIOVASCULAR problems often depends on the results of certain diagnostic tests and procedures. While you do not usually order these tests or do them, you do need to know what they are so you can prepare the patient for them both physically and psychologically. To do this you must know why a certain test is apt to be ordered and what the patient can expect during the procedure and afterward, so you can consider these things when planning the patient's care.

Here are the tests and procedures most commonly used in identifying cardiovascular disease and what you need to know about them.

Noninvasive tests first

Chest X-rays are usually among the first tests ordered when there is any reason to suspect cardiac malfunction. They are used primarily to show cardiac enlargement and pulmonary congestion. X-rays can show *pulmonary congestion* resulting from left heart failure as an opacity in the central hilar region, which fans out peripherally from the hilar region and gives the area above the base of the heart the look of "antlers."

In chronic forms of pulmonary congestion, you may see

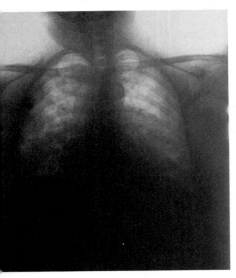

On the lookout
Conditions such as congestive
heart failure and pulmonary
edema can be diagnosed and
evaluated with chest X-rays like
the one above. Here you can see
hilar congestion and prominent
pulmonary vascular markings.
These "butterfly or bat-wing con-
figurations," as they are sometimes called, indicate congestion.
Notice, too, how enlarged
the patient's heart is.

interstitial edema as diffuse cloudiness in the central lung
fields that may resemble the shape of a butterfly. You may also
notice blunting of the costophrenic angles that reflects fluid
accumulation in these interlobular spaces. If a great deal of
fluid accumulates, you may see marked opaque lines at the
periphery or even more centrally (Kerley B or Kerley A lines).
These chest X-rays findings can detect interstitial edema even
before auscultatory findings become abnormal.

Alveolar edema appears as "cotton-puff" cloudiness in the
central lung field that spreads peripherally and superiorly as
edema in the air sacs worsens. Such accumulations of fluid
produce fine mid- to late inspiratory rales. X-ray confirms the
auscultatory findings and helps determine the extent of the
edema.

You can detect *cardiac enlargement* on chest X-rays by
estimating the cardiothoracic ratio. To get a fairly accurate
estimate, measure the diameter of the cardiac silhouette at its
widest point; then compare it to the widest diameter of the
thoracic cage. The thoracic cage should be at least twice as
wide as the heart (except on posterior-anterior [P-A] views
taken by portable X-ray). Of course, comparison with previous X-rays can greatly help in evaluating cardiac size, especially in patients with chronic lung disease. Such a patient's
heart may be quite small compared to that in a person with
normal lungs. What is cardiac enlargement for one may be
within the "normal" limits for others.

When comparing chest X-rays for cardiac enlargement, be
sure to note whether the X-ray was taken during maximum
inspiration. To get the most information from chest X-rays,
motivate the patient to take the deepest breath he can during
this test. If the patient is lethargic or confused, you may have
to call on a family member to persuade the patient to cooperate.

Standard chest X-rays are usually taken with the patient
standing upright. However, if the patient is unable to stand,
chest X-rays may be taken at the bedside. When preparing a
patient for bedside X-ray, be sure to elevate the head of the bed
as high as the patient can tolerate. This reduces the pressure of
the abdominal contents on the diaphragm and, consequently,
on the thoracic structures and allows a better X-ray.

Chest X-rays may also show *cardiac calcifications*. However, in order to determine their exact location (valvular or

subvalvular), additional tests are required.

Fluoroscopic and other tests
The cardiac fluoroscopic examination allows the examiner to see the heart from different views while it is in motion. For example, fluoroscopy of cardiac calcifications and their motion during the cardiac cycle helps to pinpoint their location. Cardiac fluoroscopy helps to evaluate wall motion and movement of prosthetic heart valves. It also identifies ventricular aneurysm (a paradoxical bulging motion of the aneurysmal sac appears during cardiac systole).

The *cardiac series* is a fluoroscopic cardiac examination in which the examiner watches the descent of swallowed barium through the esophagus from different angles. Since the esophagus is anatomically located immediately behind the heart, cardiac enlargement changes esophageal contour. Cardiac fluoroscopic examinations are given in an upright position; unlike the gastrointestinal series, they don't require the patient to fast beforehand. Many institutions avoid using fluoroscopy because it entails increased exposure to radiation. They concentrate instead on more benign techniques — usually echocardiography and electrocardiography.

Echocardiography uses ultrasound to study the location and motion of heart structures. A transducer, the size of a dime, is placed on the sternum with the tip directed towards the structures being studied. Then, ultrahigh frequency sound waves of short duration are transmitted through the transducer to these structures. The same transducer receives the echos produced as the sound waves reverberate; in turn, it relays the echos to the echocardiograph machine which records these sounds on paper.

The echos produced this way vary with the density and mobility of the structures. A trained interpreter can examine recorded echos and conclude from them information about valve leaflet mobility and position, heart wall motion during systole and diastole, and any extraneous "noises" that may be coming from intracardiac growths. Echocardiography has proven especially valuable for diagnosing atrial myxomas, ventricular aneurysms and pericardial effusions. It's also used for assessing mitral and aortic valvular dysfunction, cardiac chamber dilatation, myocardial hypertrophy, and abnormal septal wall motion.

Differentiating techniques
The two most common techniques in echocardiography are M-mode (motion-made) and two-dimensional (cross-sectional). When a detailed view of cardiac structures is desired, both techniques may be performed.

M-mode echocardiography is used to record the motion of intracardiac structures. In this method, a single rodlike ultrasound beam hits the heart, is reflected off the cardiac structures, and is then converted into electrical impulses. These impulses are displayed on a screen, and a vertical view of cardiac structures is produced.

Two-dimensional echocardiography is used to record lateral motion and provide correct spatial relationships between cardiac structures. In this technique, the ultrasound beam quickly sweeps through an arc and produces a cross-sectional or fan-shaped view of cardiac structures.

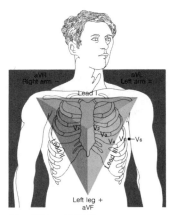

The 12-lead EKG
The 12-lead EKG uses electrodes to picture different anatomic areas of the heart and to pinpoint sites of damage. There are three groups of leads:
• *Standard limb leads* (I, II, III) simultaneously record the electrical forces of the heart as they flow toward the extremities. With these bipolar leads (two electrodes), the right arm is always the negative pole; the left leg, always positive. The left arm can be positive (in lead I) or negative (in lead III). When current flows toward the positive pole, the deflections of the EKG wave will be upright. When it flows toward the negative pole, the deflections will be inverted.
• *Unipolar augmented leads* record activity from the shoulders and the left leg and are called aVR (augmented right), aVL (augmented left), and aVF (augmented foot).
• *Precordial leads* (V_1 to V_6) record the electrical activity from six different positions on the chest. They are designated by the letter V, followed by a number.

How to prepare patients for echocardiography? Mainly, relieve their anxiety about this relatively unfamiliar procedure. Patients might expect needles, electric charges, or X-rays, but echocardiography is a painless and benign procedure. The patient merely lies flat on his back or on his left side for about 15 minutes. During this time, he may be asked to breathe in certain ways to help direct the sound waves toward the heart structures being studied.

Sometimes echocardiography and phonocardiography are combined in a procedure called echophonocardiography. This makes it possible to compare cardiac motion (obtained by echocardiograph) and the recorded cardiac sounds. It can identify the position of the valves and aortic valve leaflets during abnormal heart sounds and thus pinpoint the source of abnormal sounds. Your patient should know that during the echophonocardiography, a trained observer will be listening to his amplified heart sounds. The room must be very quiet to eliminate the recording of extraneous sounds. Just as during echocardiography, the patient may be asked to turn, lie flat, or perform specific breathing maneuvers.

EKG indispensable
Cardiovascular evaluation is incomplete without a 12-lead electrocardiogram (EKG). This graphic display of cardiac electrical activity provides invaluable data. It's one of the few diagnostic tests that you may be responsible for doing and must know how to interpret outside of an intensive care setting. To do this, you need to know the normal cardiac electrical events, including conduction and recording (see insert).

The 12-lead EKG records electrical activity from 12 universally accepted lead placements and offers a comprehensive assessment of cardiac electrical events. The 12-lead EKG offers much more information than the single lead commonly used for intensive care monitoring. Quite typically, deviations from normal occur in some leads, and not in others. If you're shopping for a car, you don't inspect it from one angle. You walk all around it. Just so, the 12-lead EKG "walks" around the heart to record its electrical phenomena from different angles.

Remember, though, that some abnormalities occur only intermittently (such as arrhythmias or ischemic disturbances). The standard 12-lead EKG records only about 70 electrical impulses out of more than 100,000 that occur in 24 hours. So, understandably, intermittent abnormalities are easily missed. Moreover, an EKG disturbance may show only when the patient has symptoms (which he may perceive as outright pain or as vague discomfort) or during exercise. For this reason, a doctor may order a 12-lead EKG to be done during an episode of chest pain (when repolarization disturbances from cardiac ischemia are most likely to show). In most cases, ischemic chest pain produces a depression in the S-T segment, an inversion of the T wave, or both S-T segment and T wave deviations. When chest pain subsides, the EKG usually reverts to normal. So, if you're testing a patient during chest pain, be sure to complete the test before giving such drugs as nitroglycerin to relieve it. Obviously, you must complete it as quickly as possible so the patient doesn't have to endure the pain any longer than necessary. Be sure to mark the tracing as one taken during chest pain.

Who needs an EKG?

Ideally, every adult should have a baseline 12-lead EKG once every 5 years. An EKG is valuable in detecting the presence and location of myocardial infarction, ischemia, conduction delay, chamber enlargement, or arrhythmias. It's also useful whenever there's any reason to expect changes from previous recordings and for monitoring electrolyte abnormalities or the effects of drugs.

The stress test (EKG during exercise) is one of the best noninvasive tools for assessing cardiac response to increased work load. This test has proven valuable in determining functional capacity after heart surgery and, after myocardial infarction (at least 14 days after the acute event), in establishing readiness for an exercise program. It's also used to identify cardiac ischemia as the source of chest discomfort. The exercise test does not require that your patient fast. However, he should not have food, cigarettes, or caffeinated beverages for 2 hours before the test.

The exercise test can be done on a special bicycle (on which the work load can be set and increased) or on treadmills with adjustable speed and grade controls. Throughout this test, the cardiogram is continuously monitored along with occasional simultaneous recordings of the patient's blood pressure response. Throughout, the patient is asked about any symptoms.

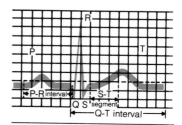

Making waves

The waves of an EKG correlate with the electrical stimulation that precedes the mechanical contraction and relaxation of the heart. These waves have arbitrarily been labeled the P, QRS, and T waves.

The P wave reflects depolarization of the atria and therefore is a good indication of SA node function. The QRS complex reflects the depolarization of the ventricles. The T wave reflects the repolarization of the ventricles. (The T wave corresponding to the repolarization of the atria isn't visible because the QRS deflection obscures it.) The mass of the ventricles is much greater than that of the atria, so the QRS and T waves are much larger than the P wave.

Occasionally, another wave, called a U wave, will appear after the T wave. The U wave may reflect electrolyte disturbances or drug influence. However, U waves may appear for *no* reason in some people.

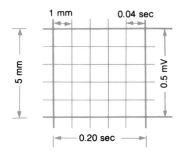

Heart blocks

In reading 12-lead EKGs, remember that the vertical lines measure the magnitude of the electrical impulse of the heart. The horizontal lines represent the time the electrical impulse takes to travel over cardiac tissue. Each small block on EKG paper is 1 mm square and represents 0.04 second. Each large box is 5 mm square and represents 0.5 mV and 0.20 second.

The test ends at the discretion of the doctor in attendance. Indications for termination of the test include any of the following: extreme fatigue, onset of angina for which the patient would normally stop activity, a drop in blood pressure, onset of arrhythmia, significant S-T changes, or attainment of desired heart rate without abnormal findings. The latter constitutes a negative test.

What constitutes a positive stress test? The criteria vary. Some institutions require S-T segment depression of 1.5 to 2 mm. In about 15% of the patients with *positive tests*, coronary artery disease cannot be documented by invasive diagnostic studies. In 15% of the patients with *negative tests*, coronary arteriography shows definite coronary artery disease. False-positive tests may result from digitalis, hypertension, or electrolyte abnormalities. If the patient is unable (because of drugs or fatigue) to exercise sufficiently to raise the heart rate to the point of stress, the test is considered nondiagnostic.

What are the contraindications for stress testing? Any recent history of unusually long or severe episodes of angina, chest pain with dyspnea, weakness, diaphoresis, nausea, or vomiting. Always check with the doctor before beginning an exercise test on a patient with any of these symptoms.

Who needs the stress test? Most doctors feel that it's indicated only for patients suspected of having ischemic heart disease, although others believe everyone over age 35 should have this test every 2 years. Lately, many health centers are using the stress test to determine physical fitness and to prescribe individual exercise programs.

Nuclear medicine

Myocardial imaging uses radioactive tracers to evaluate cardiac structures and function in much the same way as they are used for testing brain, liver, and other structures. Radioactive tracers, such as thallium and technetium pyrophosphate, attach themselves to albumin potassium or albumin potassium receptors and are easily carried by the bloodstream. Their course through the body can then be followed and recorded by scanners.

In thallium imaging, an absence of tracer material ("cold spots") indicates decreased perfusion. In technetium pyrophosphate tests, the tracer material accumulates in damaged myocardial tissue and forms a "hot spot" on the scan. Such perfusion studies can help identify acute myocardial infarction by detecting defects in myocardial perfusion or regional myocardial wall abnormalities. These tests can also be used to screen asymptomatic patients who have positive stress tests. Such patients are scanned during rest and during exercise. The test results are then compared. Radioactive tracer studies can also evaluate ventricular function. As the tracer passes through the heart chambers, it can show heart wall motion, chamber size and shape, and the percentage of blood ejected. It is important to note that these tests do not distinguish an old from a new infarction.

The patient undergoing radioactive tracer evaluation needs an intravenous infusion to carry the tracer material. Be sure to tell the patient that the amount of radioactivity used is extremely small and not harmful to himself or those near him. He will not require any special nursing care after this procedure.

Cardiac catheterization

In simple terms, cardiac catheterization is the passing of a catheter into the right or left side of the heart. Catheterization can determine blood pressure and blood flow in the chambers of the heart and allow collection of blood samples. If, during the procedure, a radiopaque dye is injected, films of the heart's ventricles (contrast ventriculography) or arteries (coronary arteriography, or angiography) can be recorded.

A patient entering a cath lab for the first time can become apprehensive unless prepared for the experience. The lab contains an overwhelming array of machinery: motion picture cameras, a fluoroscope, one or more electrocardiographs, pressure-monitoring devices, and numerous other paraphernalia. To prepare your patient, tell him that he'll be placed on a special X-ray table, virtually surrounded by equipment, some of which is even suspended from the ceiling. Once he's settled with EKG leads attached, he'll have an antecubital fossa or the groin prepped for catheter insertion. These are the sites doctors most commonly use. Sometimes, they use the axillary artery through a puncture site a few inches below the armpit. At times, the first attempt at catheter insertion is unsuccessful because of an anatomic abnormality or blockage within the target vessel. Then a second site must be used.

During the catheterization, your patient may be asked to

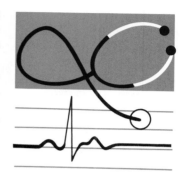

Common assessment tests for cardiac malfunction
MUSCLE DYSFUNCTION
• Chest roentgenography
• Resting 12-lead EKG
• Stress test
• Echocardiography
• Echophonocardiography
• Cardiac angiography
• Myocardial imaging

VALVULAR MALFUNCTION
• Chest roentgenography
• Resting 12-lead EKG
• Echocardiography
• Echophonocardiography
• Cardiac angiography

ELECTRICAL ABNORMALITIES
• Resting 12-lead EKG
• Ambulatory monitoring
• Stress test

CORONARY ARTERY DISEASE
• Resting 12-lead EKG
• Ambulatory monitoring
• Stress test
• Coronary angiography-arteriography
• Cardiac enzyme studies

cough or to take deep breaths. You can tell him why. Deep-breathing can facilitate catheter placement into the coronary arteries, pulmonary artery, or the wedge position. And coughing may counteract the nausea, light-headedness, or initial hypotension caused by the contrast medium (dye) and can correct arrhythmias produced by the medium's effect on the myocardium. Be sure your patient knows how to cough correctly. If hypotension persists, the patient may need treatment with a pressor agent. So, during catheterization, monitor constantly for arrhythmias and for changes in blood pressure. Also, keep handy the equipment you need for CPR and defibrillation.

Cardiac catheterization is especially helpful in evaluating....

• *Valvular heart disease*. A gradient, or difference in pressures above and below a heart valve, usually indicates this condition. Systolic pressure measurements made on both sides of a stenotic aortic valve will show a gradient across the valve. The higher the gradient, the greater the degree of stenosis. For example, left ventricular systolic pressure might measure 200 mm Hg and aortic systolic pressure only 120 mm Hg. That's an 80-mm Hg gradient across the valve. Since these pressures normally are equal, a stenosis that makes such a big difference usually requires corrective surgery.

Mitral valve disease will elevate pressures in the left atrium, hampering blood flow from the pulmonary vessels. Pressure in the pulmonary vessels (particularly the veins and capillaries) then rises to compensate for the higher atrial pressure (pulmonary hypertension).

If your patient has mitral valve disease, he may be asked to exercise (pedaling motion) during catheterization to increase venous return to his heart. The greater the degree of mitral valve disease, the higher the pressure in the pulmonary capillaries during exercise as compared with the resting pressure (which may be normal).

Incompetent valves can be visualized in ventriculography by watching retrograde flow of the contrast medium across the valve during systole.

• *Septal defects*. These defects can be evaluated by measuring blood oxygen content on each side of the abnormal septum. Elevated blood oxygen on the right indicates a left-to-right shunt at either the atrial or ventricular level. Decreased oxygen on the left indicates a right-to-left shunt.

• *Myocardial function*. Injection of contrast medium into the

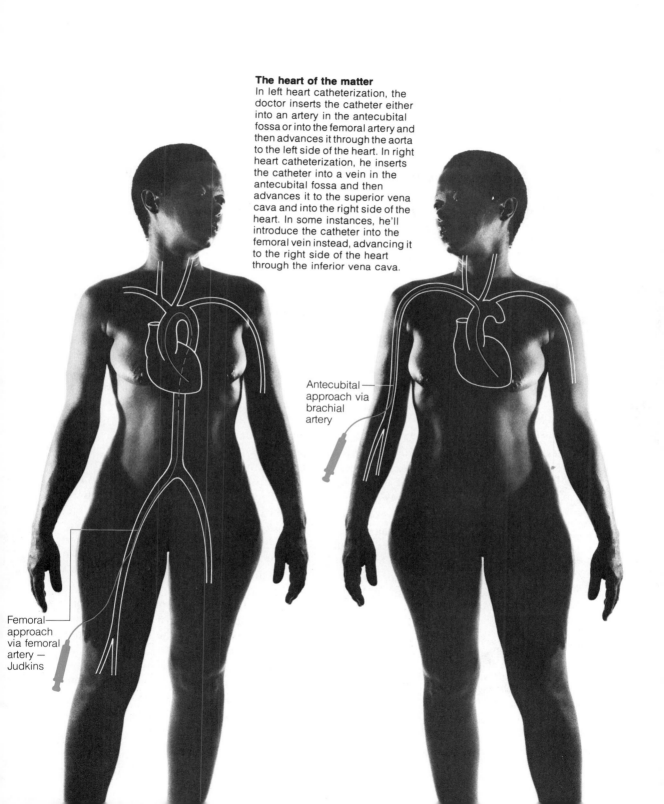

The heart of the matter
In left heart catheterization, the doctor inserts the catheter either into an artery in the antecubital fossa or into the femoral artery and then advances it through the aorta to the left side of the heart. In right heart catheterization, he inserts the catheter into a vein in the antecubital fossa and then advances it to the superior vena cava and into the right side of the heart. In some instances, he'll introduce the catheter into the femoral vein instead, advancing it to the right side of the heart through the inferior vena cava.

Antecubital approach via brachial artery

Femoral approach via femoral artery — Judkins

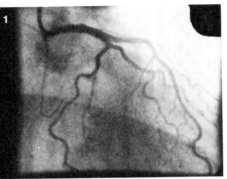

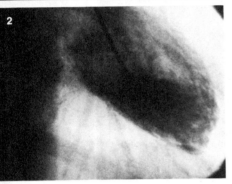

State of the heart

Cardiac catheterization includes two procedures: coronary arteriography and coronary ventriculography. For the first procedure, the patient is placed in the right anterior oblique (RAO) position. Contrast medium or dye is injected into the left coronary artery, as in figure 1. As you can see, the vessel fills completely, without narrowing or occlusion.

For ventriculography, the patient is again placed in the RAO position. During diastole, contrast medium is injected into the left ventricle. The picture that results shows wall motion, ventricular volume, the shape of the left ventricle, and the presence of any mechanical abnormalities. Figure 2 shows a normal left ventricle.

left ventricle (ventriculography) is used to assess structure and contractility of the cardiac muscle. Comparison of ventricular size during systole and diastole helps determine efficiency of muscular contraction, segmental wall motion, chamber size, and ejection fraction. The latter compares the amount of blood pumped out of the left ventricle during systole with the amount present at the end of diastole. For example, at rest, the normal left ventricle contains about 100 ml of blood. If the ventricle ejects 70 ml during systole, the ejection fraction is 70/100 (70%). In myocardial incompetence, the ejection fraction is less than 55%.

• *Wall motion.* Improper contraction of a portion of the heart chamber wall, called wall motion abnormality, commonly develops after a myocardial infarction. Such an abnormality is called hypokinesis (reduced wall motion), akinesis (absence of motion), or dyskinesis (bulging in the wall during systole).

How is this test done? Using the Sones or Judkins technique, the doctor threads a catheter (visually controlled with fluoroscopy) through an artery, advances it to the aortic root, and passes it across the aortic valve into the left ventricle. He then injects contrast medium (an opaque dye) into this area.

Arteriography: Coronary road map

Coronary arteriography, an important part of the cardiac catheterization test, produces a radiographic study of the arteries that supply the myocardium. With coronary arteriography, the doctor can clearly see the coronary arteries. Arteriography shows the sites, degree, and severity of obstruction in the coronary vessels. It allows evaluation of the size, character of blood flow, and the presence of atherosclerotic disease of vessels distal to the primary obstruction. This is an important factor in determining whether the vessel can be bypassed or if angioplasty is necessary. So, coronary arteriograms are often used to determine if a patient can benefit from surgery. Candidates for coronary bypass graft surgery must have significant lesions that can actually be bypassed. They can't be if the disease is too diffuse or if the vessel is too small to accept a graft. During evaluation for bypass, patients often receive nitroglycerin to measure its effect on the arteries and to eliminate catheter-induced spasm.

Coronary arteriography may require moving the patient from

side to side if your hospital has a stationary camera (suspended from the ceiling). A newer, nonstationary camera allows the patient to remain supine while the camera is positioned to record views of the coronary vessels from different angles.

Warn the patient to expect a feeling of flushing and warmth as the dye is injected. This is normal. Assure the patient that if he develops chest pain during the procedure, he'll receive nitroglycerin to relieve it. Tell him what other symptoms he may experience, and instruct him to let the doctor know if he experiences them. Explain that, before he goes to the cath lab, he'll be given a sedative to help him relax. But it won't put him to sleep, because his cooperation will be needed during the test procedure (taking deep breaths, turning, and so forth). Remember that your reassurance and understanding are essential to allay any fear the patient may have.

Watch for complications

Severe complications after cardiac catheterization are not common, but they can occur. The period of greatest danger is during the procedure itself when such complications as arterial occlusion from embolus, arterial spasm, acute myocardial infarction, vessel or coronary artery dissection, or perforation of the myocardium can occur. Watch for isolated premature ventricular contractions, ventricular tachycardia, and ventricular fibrillation, which can occur during or after the procedure.

If a thrombus breaks loose, or if a plaque dislodges, it can block the patient's arterial blood flow. Rarely, he may suffer a cerebrovascular accident or myocardial infarction. If the blocked vessel is an artery, your patient can lose his arterial pulse. Then the extremity itself will be white and cold. Your patient may complain of a numb feeling or severe pain.

Blood loss at the catheter insertion site is usually more profuse from arteriotomies than venotomies. If you see frank bleeding or notice swelling of the extremity at the insertion site, apply pressure to the site. The amount of pressure you apply must be greater than the pressure in the vessel. In the case of an artery, for example, the pressure applied must be greater than the systolic pressure at that site. Anytime significant bleeding occurs, whether venous or arterial, your patient's pressure will drop and his heart rate will increase. Watch for such bleeding, since even slight leakage into surrounding tissues can cause a painful hematoma. Infection at the site is

His bundle electrography
His-bundle electrography is another cardiac catheterization technique. In this test, an electrode-tipped catheter is passed into the right atrium and ventricle to record and study the activity of the heart's conduction system. For example, when an ectopic site takes over as pacemaker of the heart, the electrogram can help pinpoint the origin. The test also helps with the diagnosis of syncope, evaluates a candidate for permanent artificial pacemaker implantation, and helps select or evaluate drug therapy.

His bundle electrography is contraindicated in patients with severe coagulopathy and acute pulmonary embolism.

another potential complication. To prevent it, keep the area clean and dry. Use aseptic technique when caring for the site or changing the dressing.

After catheterization

Take vital signs frequently, as often as every 10 to 15 minutes, and record them on the patient's chart. Include blood pressure, heart rate, and pulse distal to the catheter insertion site. Check to be sure dressings are dry and intact, but not too tight. Then examine the extremity distal to the insertion site for color and warmth, and assess the quality of its pulse. Your patient will need about 6 hours of strict bed rest immediately after the test. If the femoral route was used for catheter insertion, instruct him to keep his leg extended for 6 to 8 hours; if the antecubital fossa was used, have him keep his arm extended for at least 3 hours. During this time, encourage him to wiggle his fingers and toes every half hour. Unless contraindicated, also encourage the patient to drink plenty of fluids, especially those high in potassium, to counteract the contrast medium's effect. Tell the patient that if he has pain when the local anesthetic wears off, he can have an analgesic.

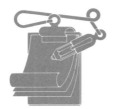

Remember these important points when preparing a patient for diagnostic testing:
1. Be aware that chest X-rays help detect pulmonary congestion and cardiac enlargement and may show cardiac calcifications.
2. Keep in mind that an EKG disturbance may be revealed only when the patient has symptoms or during exercise.
3. Know the difference in echocardiography techniques: M-mode records the motion of intracardiac structures; two-dimensional records lateral motion and provides correct spatial relationships between cardiac structures.
4. Emphasize to your patient the importance of deep breathing and coughing during cardiac catheterization in preventing nausea and light-headedness.
5. Following cardiac catheterization, closely monitor your patient for signs of complications, such as myocardial infarction, arrhythmias, cardiac tamponade, shock, and infection.

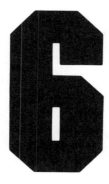

Hypertension
Risk factor in atherosclerosis

BY ROSEMARY JARLATH MALONEY, BSN, MSN

IF YOU MANAGE hypertensive patients at all, you know that the worst problem is getting them to stick to their prescribed regimen. They typically miss appointments, forget to take their medications, and neglect their diet. If they'd only cooperate, they would be much better off and you could feel better about their treatment. All too often they don't. Some sources suggest that only 13% of hypertensive patients seem to be under good control.

How can you help?

Often, patients with hypertension don't cooperate because they don't understand how hypertension is threatening their lives. You can help them to understand. First, you must understand hypertension quite well yourself.

What is hypertension? The American Heart Association, recognizing that it's different things in different people, simply calls it an *unstable or persistent elevation of pressure above the normal range*. And they estimate that more than 26 million people in the U.S. and Canada suffer from it. *That's one in every six adults*.

The prevalence among women is 3% to 4% higher than

Probable causes of hypertension

According to 1978 estimates of the American Heart Association, among people 20 years old and over, 13% of white males and 25% of black males, 17% of white females and 28% of black females have hypertension. Hypertension may be a primary or secondary disorder. This chart shows you at a glance the diagnostic possibilities according to age of onset. For example, you can see that as a person ages, the possibility of developing renal parenchymal disease or aortic coarctation decreases while the possibility of developing primary aldosteronism or essential hypertension increases. People of all ages are susceptible to pheochromocytoma.
Understanding these trends will help you assess your patient.

- ▬ ▬ Renal arterial disease
- ◥◣◥ Renal parenchymal disease
- ▬▬▬ Aortic coarctation
- ▬▬▬ Pheochromocytoma
- ▬ ▬ Essential hypertension
- ◣◥◣ Primary aldosteronism

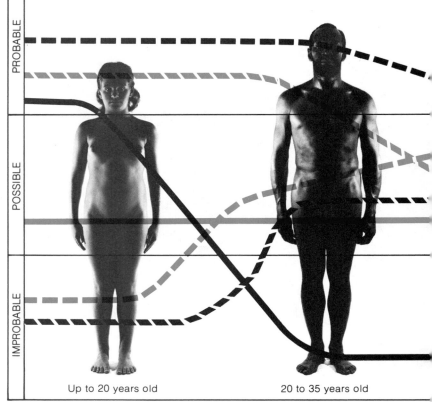

PROBABLE — POSSIBLE — IMPROBABLE

Up to 20 years old   20 to 35 years old

among men; among blacks, 11% to 12% higher than among whites (see above). Target organs — those chiefly affected — are brain, eyes, heart, and kidneys. Early symptoms? Typically, there aren't any. Or the victim may have morning headache. But the damage can go on just the same as the pressure rises.

Why blood pressure varies

Blood pressure is the relationship between a given amount and flow of fluid, the blood, and the size and tension of its container, the vessel walls. Its purpose, of course, is to perfuse even the remotest tissue with life-giving oxygen carried by the circulating red blood cells. But there are numerous variables in the two factors, blood flow and vasculature. Hence the variations in pressure.

Variables are these. The quantity of blood flow in a given time, cardiac output, is determined by: ventricular filling (partly based on plasma volume); the heart's contractility; the heart rate (primarily controlled by the autonomic nervous system); and, total peripheral vascular resistance. Peripheral vascular resistance itself depends on the caliber and tone of the

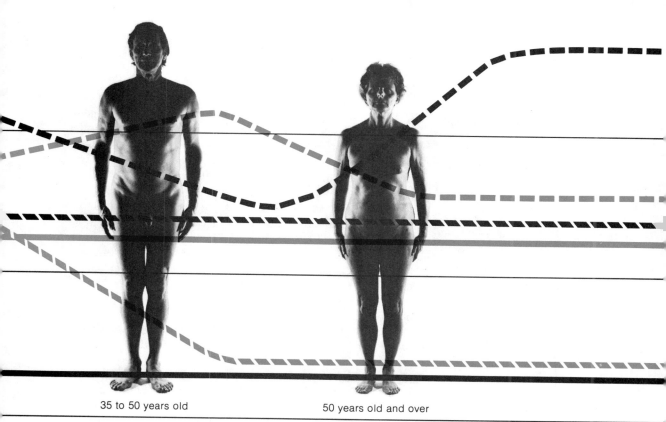

35 to 50 years old   50 years old and over

arteries, arterioles, and veins. Unless the vessels are largely occluded by atherosclerosis or some other mechanical blockage, their capacity is powerfully regulated by humoral and neural stimulation also coming from the autonomic nervous system.

Humoral agents, such as angiotensin, catecholamines, serotonin, histamine, prostaglandins, and aldosterone influence the size of the blood vessels and blood volume (by regulating sodium and water balance). Neural control is even quicker and more efficient; witness the "fight or flight" reaction to stress.

Hypertension can be controlled by manipulating almost any one of these factors, as modern pharmacological agents do. First, though, you must know what's causing it.

Classification of hypertension falls into essential and secondary. *Essential* hypertension — about 80% to 90% of all cases — has no proven cause. One theory says it's caused by increased peripheral vascular resistance coming from degenerative constriction of the arterioles. This resistance produces renal ischemia which, in turn, stimulates the renin-angiotensin and aldosterone cycles.

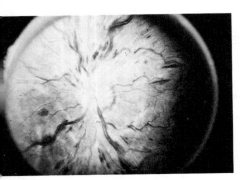

What meets the eye
This eye ground, of a 43-year-old woman, shows Grade III changes in the retina. The patient had malignant hypertension, blurred vision, papilledema of the left disc, fresh hemorrhage, and impending vein occlusion.

The remaining cases of hypertension stem from secondary causes, such as renovascular disease; pheochromocytoma; Cushing's syndrome; dysfunctions of the thyroid, pituitary, or parathyroid glands; or neurologic disorders. Primary aldosteronism is another secondary cause. It produces hypervolemia by inducing an excess reabsorption of sodium and water.

Although hypertension can occur at any age, even during childhood, essential hypertension usually occurs between the ages of 30 and 40. Common risk factors? Often, race (more common in blacks than in people of other races), stress, obesity, high dietary intake of saturated fats or sodium, use of tobacco or oral contraceptives, sedentary life-style, and aging. Also familial predisposition: siblings of known hypertensives have an added susceptibility to the disorder.

The role of stress? Because stress, anger, and frustration momentarily drive the blood pressure up, stress has been implicated as a principal factor in keeping it there. The problem is that, eventually, relieving the stress often doesn't lower the blood pressure. But, indeed, implicating stress are these facts: black men in high-stress situations have a higher incidence of hypertension than any other group; and people in societies undergoing change have a higher incidence than those in stable populations. Although arterial pressure tends to increase with advancing age in most societies, studies of Pacific island natives and Brazilian Indians have shown that such people escape hypertension as a natural consequence of aging.

Diagnostic clues

You can often assess a patient's cardiovascular status by whether he has dyspnea, orthopnea, or chest pain. Dependent edema would indicate failure of cardiac venous return, probably from right-sided heart failure. Nocturia could mean kidney involvement or heart failure. Nocturia occurs as a result of recumbency at night (increased perfusion of the renal bed enhances filtration and excretion).

If the patient has nephrosclerosis along with hypertension, proteinuria would result from the increased renal arteriolar permeability. Uremia is seldom seen in a patient with benign essential hypertension, but it is one of the hallmarks of the relentless, progressive form of the disease known as maligant hypertension. Papilledema (edema of the optic disk) is pathognomonic of malignant hypertension, and it's often accompanied by renal and cerebral symptoms. In benign essential hypertension, the early morning headache often reported in the beginning may be succeeded by fatigue, diminished mental acuity, forgetfulness, and irritability, brought on by "small strokes" — minor cerebrovascular accidents.

Examining the optic fundi gives perhaps the best information about the severity and duration of the hypertensive process. Usually, mild hypertensive retinopathy can be seen as constriction of the vessels of the eyegrounds. If you see soft exudates, hemorrhages, and papilledema, they lend an ominous prognosis. End-stage retinopathy is reflected by venous destruction and arterial obliteration, that is, the vessels thicken enough to close the intimal lumen. Unfortunately, these arteriosclerotic changes are irreversible.

Cardiac disease itself can either produce or result from the hypertensive process. Either way, cardiac involvement is the leading cause of death in hypertensive patients. So, assessment in hypertensive patients always includes thorough auscultation for changes in heart sounds (see Chapter 4).

Lab work should include some or all of these tests:
• Chest film to show cardiac size and pulmonary vasculature.
• Blood urea nitrogen (BUN) and serum creatinine to measure renal excretory function.
• Protein excretion in the urine measured over a 24-hour period, which shouldn't total more than 0.2 to 0.4 gram; if higher, it indicates renal parenchymal disease.
• Serum electrolytes, especially potassium levels (which inversely denote the secretory levels of aldosterone) since that hormone saves sodium by wasting potassium and hydrogen ions in the renal tubule.
• EKG to check for left ventricular hypertrophy characteristic of hypertensive heart disease.

Treatment goals

Treatment of hypertension aims to reduce arterial pressure and arrest atherosclerosis and progressive arteriolar disease. Most doctors consider cardiovascular risk reduced when diastolic readings are maintained at less than 90 mm Hg. This can be accomplished in up to 85% of patients.

Three kinds of drugs are used to lower blood pressure:
1. Diuretics act by promoting water and sodium excretion,

What is hypertensive crisis?

An acute rise in blood pressure (diastolic usually over 120 mm Hg). Thickening and narrowing of arterioles lead to damage of vital organs. *What precipitates it* in some hypertensive patients?
• abrupt discontinuation of antihypertensive medications
• increased salt consumption
• increased production of renin, epinephrine, and norepinephrine
• increased stress.

Therapy aims:
To lower blood pressure rapidly to prevent hypertensive encephalopathy by use of vasodilators, I.V. (nitroprusside, diazoxide, hydralazine) and sympathetic blockers (methyldopa, phentolamine, reserpine). Trimethaphan camsylate blocks both sympathetic and parasympathetic nervous systems.

Nursing responsibilities:
• Take baseline vital signs and monitor frequently: blood pressure readings from both arms, apical pulse, respirations, and temperature. Check pupils for reaction to light; assess level of consciousness and orientation to time, place, person.
• Check for dehydration. Remember, giving vasodilators to dehydrated patients can cause dangerous hypotension.
• Obtain a patient history.
• Be supportive to patient and family.
• Monitor drug therapy to prevent severe hypotension or toxic reactions.
• Teach patient and family as soon as possible about: drugs, diet, activities, avoidance of stress, and how to take home blood pressures.

Secondary hypertension

The following disorders can cause secondary hypertension, so watch for the physical findings that accompany each.

COARCTATION OF AORTA — absence of femoral pulses, decreased blood pressure in legs, weight loss, intercostal bruits

PHEOCHROMOCYTOMA — severe headache with palpitation, hypermetabolic state, elevated fasting blood sugar

PRIMARY ALDOSTERONISM — elevated blood pressure, weakness, nocturia, polydipsia, tetany, headache, numbness, hypokalemia

CUSHING'S SYNDROME — moon face, "buffalo" hump, edema

RENOVASCULAR HYPERTEN-ION — edema, hyponatremia, decreased urine output, bruit over renal artery

GLOMERULONEPHRITIS — sodium and water retention, oliguria, dyspnea, pulmonary edema, uremic odor, myocardial hypertrophy

thereby reducing plasma volume and intraarterial sodium.

2. Sympatholytics diminish the sympathetic reflexes that produce a stepped-up heart rate and blood pressure.

3. Vasodilators relax the arterial smooth-muscle walls.

The drug chosen in each case depends on what's causing the patient's hypertension. Although antihypertensive drugs are used in combination in most cases, they are usually begun singly. If the patient's diastolic pressure is consistently above 90, treatment almost always begins with a diuretic. If, after a trial period of 1 to 2 months, more control is needed, the next therapeutic step would include reserpine (Serpasil) or methyldopa (Aldomet).

If the second drug added to the diuretic doesn't adequately reduce blood pressure, a third drug will be added — most likely hydralazine (Apresoline). If a patient's hypertension is traceable to a high renin secretion, then a beta blocker — propranolol (Inderal) — may be used instead of a diuretic from the outset. Recently, beta blockers have also proven to be effective as second-line antihypertensive agents when combined with a diuretic or as first-line agents when given without a diuretic.

New agents for long-term management of hypertension have helped minimize disturbing side effects. Clonidine hydrochloride (Catapres), an adrenergic inhibitor, acts on the cardiorespiratory center in the brain's medulla. By stimulating alpha-adrenergic receptor sites centrally, it inhibits sympathetic outflow. Peripheral effects of this drug are diminished vasoconstriction and decreased peripheral vascular resistance. Prazosin (Minipress) relaxes peripheral arterioles and decreases total peripheral vascular resistance. The search continues for the "ideal" agent. Good control of elevated blood pressure is indispensable in forestalling cumulative target-organ damage and avoiding hypertensive crisis.

Patient education crucial

Your hypertensive patient needs painstaking education if he's to avoid a worsening illness and repeated hospital admission. Only if he understands his disease can he accept and respond with purpose to a treatment plan that seems superfluous to a patient without distressing symptoms.

So, always explain the pathology of hypertension and its ramifications. You've got to convince the patient that he has a lifelong illness that needs controlling, *even if he doesn't feel bad*. Ideally, include a family member when you are planning and explaining treatment. This will gain the patient greater understanding and support at home.

Then, find out how well the patient himself understands his disease, and what makes it worse. Discuss general principles of healthful living — weight control, diet, daily habits, minimizing stress. Does he understand that sodium restriction reduces blood volume and lightens the work of the heart? Does he know that caffeine is a powerful vasoconstrictor and increases the work of the heart? Does he know that coffee, tea, and cola drinks (and some ordinary medications such as Anacin tablets) all contain caffeine? Does he know that nicotine acts much like caffeine? Make sure he knows these reasons why he'll be told to give up certain things.

Patients with hypertension also need to avoid what stress they can, or learn to handle it differently. Various techniques for mitigating stress have been successful: prayer, psychotherapy, yoga, and biofeedback among them.

What about side effects?
If the patient knows what to expect, you can save him a lot of worry. For example, warn men that failure to ejaculate is commonplace with guanethidine (Ismelin) and other agents that decrease sympathetic outflow. (See Appendices for common antihypertensive drugs, their dosages, and common side effects.)

One of the most troublesome, even dangerous, effects is excessive potassium loss from diuretic therapy. This can be intensified by combining diuretics with other drugs such as corticosteroids. The first sign of it may be calf pain or leg cramps. Or the patient may complain of weakness and fatigue. To keep track of it, the doctor will order occasional checks of the patient's serum potassium level. If he doesn't order a potassium supplement, recommend foods high in potassium: orange juice, bananas, apricots, figs, raisins, meat, leafy green vegetables, and seafood. If salt is restricted but not forbidden, you may suggest Lite-Salt, a combination of sodium and potassium chloride.

In patients taking high doses of thiazide or furosemide (Lasix), serum uric acid is commonly elevated. Explain this to any patient with joint problems. Gouty symptoms can easily

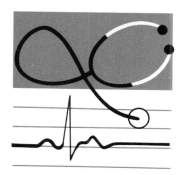

Diagnostic profile
Blood pressure consistently
  above 140/90
Anginal pain
Edema of the extremities
Dyspnea on exertion
Retinal hemorrhages and
  exudates
Severe occipital headaches with
  nausea and vomiting,
  drowsiness, anxiety, and
  mental impairment
Late signs of associated arteriolar
  nephrosclerosis: polyuria,
  nocturia, protein and red blood
  cells in urine

be controlled with allopurinol (Zyloprim).

You can help with the medication schedule. The patient's doctor sets the medication schedule, but there may be much you can do to make it more acceptable or easily followed. For example, suppose the prescription says twice a day. What does twice a day mean? First thing in the morning and last thing at night, even if he gets up at 6 a.m. and goes to bed at 2 a.m.? How can he space the doses better and still be sure of remembering his medication? Let him offer you some suggestions. *If it's his idea, he'll be more likely to follow it.*

While you're trying to impress your patient with the need for sticking to his program and coming back for regular review, be sure to cover his whole treatment program thoroughly. Explain each of his medications and their purposes.

Home blood pressure measurement? For the patients who will use it meaningfully, home blood pressure measurement can be a great help in guiding therapy. Usually, they can get truer readings when relaxed at home than when tense about the possible results in the nurse's or doctor's office. You have to use your judgment about which patients to enlist in a home measurement program. Or select a member of the family to do the job. And emphasize that it isn't the single reading that counts, but the trend.

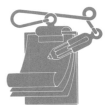

Remember these important points when managing a patient with hypertension:

1. Consider a family history of hypertension, stress, obesity, high dietary intake of saturated fats or sodium, use of tobacco or oral contraceptives, sedentary life-style, and aging as key risk factors in essential hypertension.

2. Be aware that secondary causes of hypertension include renovascular disease; pheochromocytoma; primary aldosteronism; Cushing's syndrome; dysfunction of the thyroid, pituitary, or parathyroid glands; and neurologic disorders.

3. Examine the optic fundi for clues to hypertension's severity and duration.

4. Familiarize yourself with antihypertensive drugs: diuretics, sympatholytics, and vasodilators.

5. Emphasize to your patient that hypertension is a lifelong illness that needs controlling, even if he is asymptomatic.

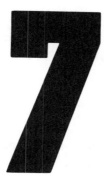

7

Coronary Artery Disease
Stages of progression

BY CHRISTINE W. CANNON, RN, MSN

WE'RE QUITE USED TO TREATING the end stage of coronary artery disease — myocardial infarction — vigorously and effectively. With the latest techniques, we can terminate ventricular fibrillation and even resuscitate after cardiac arrest. But we don't do nearly as much for patients in earlier stages of coronary artery disease. Do we ignore these earlier stages simply because they generally produce no symptoms? Or because doing something meaningful about them is much more difficult? In either case, we're not doing as much as we can.

We can do more

The most important thing we can do is help patients prevent the onset of coronary artery disease. And that's quite a challenge. The ultimate cause of coronary artery disease is still unknown, and the meaning of and methods for controlling risk factors (such as cholesterol) keep changing with ongoing scientific study. Moreover, many of the risk factors (smoking, eating habits, personality factors) are quite difficult to change, even with others' strong support. You can't guarantee that the patient will escape further illness even if he does *everything* you suggest. Despite all this, we've got to routinely

Controllable factors in C.A.D.

Hypertension greatly predisposes to coronary artery disease. As diastolic blood pressure exceeds 90 mm Hg and the systolic exceeds 140 mm Hg, the risk of coronary artery disease increases sharply. In uncontrolled hypertension, the heart must work harder to force blood from the left ventricle into the constricted peripheral circuit. Consequently, the myocardium hypertrophies, needing much more oxygen to energize the greater muscle mass of the left ventricle. Controlling blood pressure requires control of obesity, restricted salt intake, and the careful use of diuretics and antihypertensives. Uncontrolled hypertension commonly results from late diagnosis or poor compliance with recommended treatment.

Diabetes is another source of circulatory damage. Controlling it through diet and insulin aims to reduce connective tissue degeneration, which may accelerate atherogenesis; and to regulate body insulin, which may affect lipid metabolism and arterial response.

Diet may affect one risk factor, hyperlipidemia. High levels of cholesterol, triglyceride, and saturated fatty acids have been linked with increased coronary artery disease. We can recommend moderation in daily fat intake (using more polyunsaturated fats than saturated) and control of obesity. Probably the best answer is to encourage regular, vigorous physical activity to use up those ingested fats.

Smoking overstimulates the heart, constricts peripheral blood vessels, and releases carbon monoxide which interferes with myocardial oxygenation.

teach patients with coronary artery disease (CAD):

- what we know about the process of atherosclerosis
- what risk factors are and how to control them
- how to recognize, relieve, and prevent anginal attacks.

Group teaching ideal

Teaching such patients in groups helps them learn that other people share the same problems. Group discussions encourage free expression of some of the anxiety, depression, and denial common in such patients. In groups, patients can swap ideas and methods for making difficult adjustments (like tips for reducing stress and stopping smoking) — a real plus for patients struggling to control their disease by changing their life-style.

What information should *you* provide? Begin with a simple explanation of the structure and function of the heart (with emphasis on the coronary arteries). Be sure to include signs and symptoms of coronary artery disease; risk factors and how to control them; diet management; coping with stress; therapeutic exercise; and control of smoking habits. Offer helpful pamphlets such as those from the American Heart Association. You may want to make personal visits or phone calls to persons who have special problems or need special instructions.

Risk factors: Some controllable — some not

You're surely familiar with the relationship between certain "risk factors" and coronary artery disease. Risk factors are usually classified as uncontrollable (age, sex, race, and heredity) and controllable (diabetes, hypertension, hyperlipidemia, sedentary lifestyle, smoking, and stress). When teaching patients about risk factors, it's best to emphasize the controllable ones. This offers the patient hope that he *can* feel better, and something he can do to make it happen. But resist the temptation to overstate the amount of control that's attainable. For example, diet has been proclaimed the answer to one risk factor, hyperlipidemia, and low-fat, low-cholesterol diets have become popular even though some question the link between dietary habits and serum cholesterol levels. Actually, a strict low-fat diet decreases serum cholesterol by less than 10% of its baseline level, because the body synthesizes its own cholesterol. New evidence suggests that high cholesterol levels may

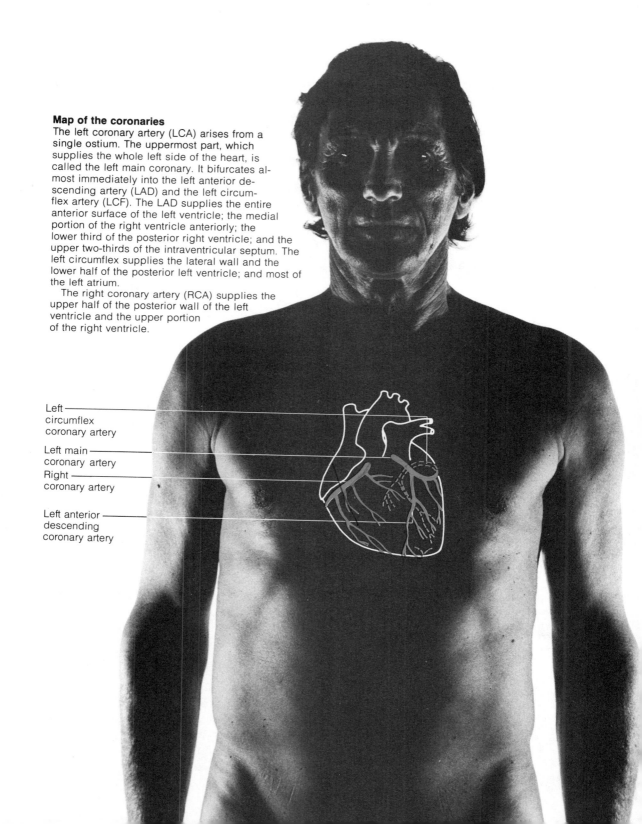

Map of the coronaries
The left coronary artery (LCA) arises from a single ostium. The uppermost part, which supplies the whole left side of the heart, is called the left main coronary. It bifurcates almost immediately into the left anterior descending artery (LAD) and the left circumflex artery (LCF). The LAD supplies the entire anterior surface of the left ventricle; the medial portion of the right ventricle anteriorly; the lower third of the posterior right ventricle; and the upper two-thirds of the intraventricular septum. The left circumflex supplies the lateral wall and the lower half of the posterior left ventricle; and most of the left atrium.

The right coronary artery (RCA) supplies the upper half of the posterior wall of the left ventricle and the upper portion of the right ventricle.

Left circumflex coronary artery

Left main coronary artery

Right coronary artery

Left anterior descending coronary artery

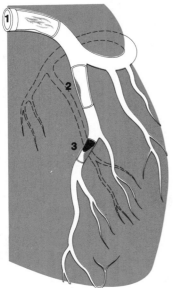

Hard-hearted
Atherosclerosis causes 90% of all coronary artery disease. The remaining 10% is caused by congenital defects in the coronary vascular system, dissecting aneurysms, infectious vasculitis, or syphilis.

Coronary artery disease develops through three progressive stages. 1) In childhood, fatty streaks appear in the arteries — thin, smooth, slightly elevated yellow dots or lines that, in some cases, regress completely. 2) Fibrous plaques develop, reflecting both a low-grade inflammatory reaction and a healing response. This stage usually indicates that the disease will progress further. 3) Complications develop: necrosis, calcification, and vascularization with or without hemorrhage into the plaque. Such changes predispose the patient to thrombosis.

actually result from impaired conversion of cholesterol into bile acid. This conversion may be affected by certain noxious chemicals (such as carbon monoxide) prevalent in industrialized countries.

What can we reasonably recommend to patients with hyperlipidemia? We can recommend moderation in daily fat intake (using more polyunsaturated fats); control of obesity (obesity increases body synthesis of cholesterol); and regular, vigorous physical activity to use up the ingested fats. Regular exercise offers many proven benefits: reduction in heart rate, systolic blood pressure, blood lipids, and body weight; and increases in exercise tolerance, cardiac efficiency, fibrinolytic activity, and overall well-being. But don't *promise* the patient that if he exercises regularly all will be well. It may not. There's always one patient in the cardiac rehabilitation class who announces that he had a myocardial infarction even though he watched his diet and jogged regularly for the last 10 years.

What can you tell patients about stress? No one can totally avoid it. But patients can learn to reduce it by avoiding noise and crowds; by changing stressful jobs; by learning to accept what cannot be changed; by exercising to release tension (yoga, walking, or just deep-breathing exercises); by getting adequate rest and sleep; and by developing an enjoyable hobby.

Know the uncontrollable factors

Coronary artery disease is more prevalent in whites than in blacks; in men than in women; and in middle-aged and older people than in young people (although fatty streaks in the intimal arterial layer, the precursors of occluding plaques, can be found in the young). Women seem to escape coronary artery disease until after menopause, probably because of a retarding influence of estrogen on atherogenesis. But the incidence of coronary artery disease does seem to be rising among premenopausal women, especially among those who take oral contraceptives, smoke, or work at competitive, stress-producing jobs.

Familial tendency toward coronary artery disease seems a strong risk factor. Many young coronary patients had fathers, brothers, or grandfathers with premature coronary artery disease. No one can change his age, race, or hereditary disposition. But knowing the potential effects may motivate the high-risk candidate to control the factors he *can* change.

Recognize the coronary-prone patient

Let's consider Mr. Stern, a 48-year-old accountant. His father and brother both had died prematurely of coronary disease. But Mr. Stern liked to boast that he'd never been sick a day in his life. He loved the challenges of tax time — the phone calls, the appointments, the deadlines and, most of all, the competition with the younger accountants in his office. He smoked 3 packs of cigarettes a day to "help him relax," and boasted that he could eat almost anything — and usually did. He was 40 pounds overweight. Recently, he'd been having frequent sudden, short attacks of pressure-like "indigestion." He noticed this often while rushing back to his office after lunch, sometimes while working at his desk, and sometimes during sexual intercourse.

You won't be surprised to know that his "indigestion" was actually angina pectoris, his first warning that coronary artery disease was gradually cutting off the blood supply to his heart muscle. During cardiac evaluation studies, Mr. Stern was given a submaximal exercise stress test. He developed his typical "indigestion" after 3 minutes on the treadmill. At the same time, he developed S-T segment depression of 2 mm and S-T straightening (a positive stress test for CAD). His resting EKG appeared normal, but his resting blood pressure was 150/98. His serum cholesterol was high at 300 mg %.

What is angina?

Angina is the discomfort caused by inadequate delivery of oxygen to the myocardium (myocardial ischemia). The resulting accumulation of acid metabolites stimulates myocardial nerve endings to transmit pain to the cardiac nerves and upper thoracic posterior roots (which explains why patients can feel cardiac pain in the left shoulder and arm). Typically, the patient describes anginal pain as a sudden and transient discomfort in the anterior chest. It's brought on by exertion and relieved by rest.

Angina is not always easy to diagnose because of the varying character of the pain. But if you ask the right questions, you should be able to identify probable anginal pain. Your questions should always include these:

- Where is the pain? Point to it.
- Describe the pain: What does it feel like?
- How did it start? What brings it on? What relieves it?

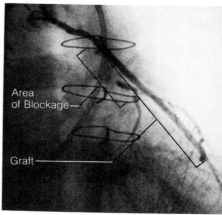

Area of Blockage—

Graft——

Change of heart
In this coronary angiogram, you can see an occlusion of the anterior descending coronary artery, which prevented distal filling until a graft was inserted to bypass the occlusion. Grafts like this are formed by taking a vein segment (usually part of the saphenous), inverting it, and anastomosing it above and below the occlusion.

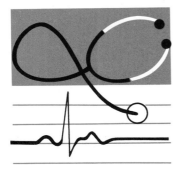

Diagnostic profile for angina
EKG abnormalities during and
after exercise
● Chest X-rays
● Cardiac catheterization
before surgery
● Nitroglycerin will shorten an
attack of anginal pain or increase
the tolerance to exercise.

STABLE ANGINA: occurs over a
long time in same pattern of onset,
duration, and intensity of
symptoms.

UNSTABLE ANGINA: frequency,
intensity, and duration of
symptoms increase as
atherosclerotic process
progresses. About 50% of
patients will infarct within 3 to 18
months after onset.

PRINZMETAL'S ANGINA: chest
discomfort at rest due to coronary
artery spasm causes transient S-T
segment elevation and pain.

ANGINA DECUBITUS: chest
discomfort that occurs in the
recumbent position, relieved by
sitting or standing.

NOCTURNAL ANGINA: occurs only
at night, but not necessarily in the
recumbent position.

INTRACTABLE ANGINA: chronic
chest discomfort that is physically
incapacitating, and refractory to
medical treatment.

● Does the pain seem to move? Where?
● Have you had the same pain before? How long did it last?
● Do you have any other symptoms or discomfort? (Look for signs of shortness of breath, profuse sweating, and nausea.)

Classically, anginal pain occurs substernally with radiation down the left arm and lasts 3 to 5 minutes. Patients describe it as heavy, squeezing, constricting, choking, smothering, expanding, aching, or burning; some simply say "something's not right in my chest." Some patients just can't seem to find the right words, so watch for nonverbal clues as well. A grimace with a fist clenched against the sternum is one reliable nonverbal clue. You can almost count on angina pectoris when you see it.

Anginal pain usually occurs during exertion, emotional stress, isometric exercises, and stressful dream states. It's especially likely when the patient is cold or digesting a meal. Other factors that can bring on an anginal attack include anger, fright, and strong emotion — all of which increase myocardial oxygen consumption. Remember that oxygen needs are chronically exaggerated in aortic valve disease accompanied by left ventricular hypertrophy, obesity, hypertension, anemia, hyperthyroidism, and hypoxemia. Anginal pain may radiate to the neck, jaw, shoulder, elbow, down the arm — especially the left — or even to the fingers. Remember that patients with angina pectoris need not describe their pain in classic terms, and they can feel such pain anywhere between the jaw and epigastrium.

Chest pain: Anginal or not?
Chest pain may signal a variety of disorders, but your first concern is always to decide whether or not the pain is anginal. Always ask the patient:

● *Is the pain better or worse when you breathe in or out?* Anginal pain isn't affected by respiration.

● *Is the pain better or worse when you change your body positions?* Again, anginal pain usually isn't affected by position changes.

While the pain of angina and myocardial infarction is unaffected by changes in position, the pain of pericarditis often decreases when the patient sits of leans forward; it may increase when he lies on his left side, laughs, or coughs.

● *Does the pain seem deep or superficial; mild or intense?*

Cardiac pain seems deep and unusually intense; noncardiac pain is typically described as mild "soreness" or dull aching.

• *Can you point to the pain with one finger?* Cardiac pain tends to be diffuse, not sharply localized.

If you're present during an actual anginal attack, your assessment should include physical signs, vital signs, and an EKG. The patient may look normal but, more likely, obviously distressed. Generally, he looks quite pale and has cool, damp skin. His pulse and blood pressure may be elevated, especially if the angina comes on after exertion. In some patients examined during an actual attack of angina, you may hear an atrial gallop (S_4). In some patients, you can detect these vibrations only when the patient is in the left lateral position. Some patients have ventricular gallop (S_3), suggesting a temporary decompensation of the left ventricle. In some, the S_3 and S_4 sounds may merge to form a summation gallop.

Your responsibility to a patient with angina includes prompt action to relieve pain. Help the patient into a comfortable resting position (with his head elevated) and give oxygen. The patient with confirmed angina needs a sublingual nitroglycerin tablet at the first hint of pain and another one at 5-minute intervals if pain persists. The doctor may request an EKG during the pain episode — before administering nitroglycerin. Stay with your patient until the attack subsides.

Between attacks, the patient should keep a few nitroglycerin tablets with him at all times and at his bedside (in a tightly closed, dark glass bottle). He can then take them as needed to relieve or prevent angina. If the pain is not relieved by three nitroglycerin tablets taken at 5-minute intervals, instruct him to call the doctor or go to the hospital's emergency department. Warn the patient that nitroglycerin may cause reflex tachycardia, a pounding headache, flushing, and occasional dizziness. And warn against standing for about 30 minutes after taking it (and standing up *suddenly* thereafter).

Of course, preventing an attack is always better than dealing with one after it happens. So, you must help patients identify those activities that trigger angina. For Mr. Stern, trigger activities included any exercise (walking, sexual intercourse) soon after meals and stress, usually accompanied by cigarette smoking. He was encouraged to relax whenever he felt the demands of his work were "getting to him," to go outside and deeply breathe some fresh air for 5 to 10 minutes. He was

HDL: New heart-risk key

A new lab test predictive of coronary artery disease measures serum high-density lipoproteins (HDL) in conjunction with serum cholesterol levels. HDL, it appears, inhibits the entry of cholesterol into arterial cells. It also increases the rate at which cholesterol leaves the cells.

A cholesterol:HDL ratio of 5 reflects a "standard" risk; of 10 doubles the risk; and of 20 triples the risk, with a likelihood of triple-vessel coronary artery disease. A desirable ratio is 3:5 or less.

When considered alone, an HDL level of 45 mg/100 ml in men and 55 mg/100 ml in women is standard. (The higher HDL levels in women may reflect their lesser predisposition to coronary artery disease.) Preventive care now involves raising HDL levels (largely through exercise) as much as lowering total serum cholesterol.

Haste makes waste
Cardiologists have identified a personality type (Type A) that's especially vulnerable to acute myocardial infarctions. This person has a malignant compulsion to achieve as much as possible in as little time as possible.

The following physiologic changes are found in a Type A person: increased secretion of catecholamines; high fasting levels of triglycerides, beta lipoproteins, and cholesterol; faster blood clotting; and slow clearance of fat from the blood. These physiologic changes reverse with behavior modification.

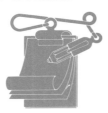

advised he could prevent angina during intercourse by getting into better physical condition with regular, prescribed exercise and by using nitroglycerin just before. To reduce his baseline myocardial oxygen requirements, Mr. Stern needed to reduce his weight and blood pressure and to stop smoking.

Mr. Stern's drug regimen included vasodilation with a long-acting nitroglycerin (Nitro-Dur) patch applied to a hairless chest site once daily. He could augment the long-acting nitroglycerin with sublingual nitroglycerin for rapid onset. Sublingual nitroglycerin has a short duration of action, so it may need to be repeated once or twice every 5 minutes during an anginal attack. Mr. Stern also took atenolol (Tenormin), 50 mg once a day to reduce myocardial oxygen demands by decreasing heart rate and contractility and blood pressure.

Remember these important points when caring for a patient with CAD:
1. Help patients with CAD understand atherosclerosis; identify and control possible risk factors; and recognize, relieve, and prevent anginal attacks.
2. When teaching a patient about risk factors, emphasize that some factors are controllable to offer him hope for improved health.
3. Although CAD is most prevalent in men, be aware that among women, those who smoke, take oral contraceptives, and work in high-stress-level jobs have a higher incidence of CAD.
4. Know how to differentiate anginal (generalized soreness) pain from chest pain (sharp, centralized).
5. Watch for the patient whose personality predisposes him to CAD: he's impatient, competitive, and fearful of wasting time.

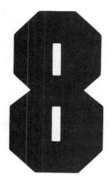

Acute Myocardial Infarction
The ultimate obstruction

BY CATHERINE CIAVERELLI MANZI, RN

YOU'VE JUST TAKEN A CALL from the rescue squad. They're on their way with a middle-aged man who collapsed on the street. Their tentative diagnosis: acute myocardial infarction. Do you feel competent to cope? Do you know what physical changes to expect? What symptoms to look for and what they mean? What lab data will be pertinent and how to interpet the results? What complications are possible and how to guard against them? And, of course, what treatment is likely to be used so you can be ready to give it promptly?

If you can confidently answer *yes* to all these questions, the care you give patients with acute myocardial infarction (AMI) is quite possibly lifesaving. But if you can't, you may find this review helpful.

Chest pain typical

Patients with an AMI usually have severe chest pain, which differs from that of angina pectoris in that it lasts longer than 20 minutes. Most angina subsides in only a few minutes. The pain of AMI usually persists from a half hour to several hours; rarely, it may last no longer than 5 minutes. Such pain or discomfort may begin anytime, during exercise, rest, or sleep.

What happens in AMI

As you know, when atherosclerosis narrows or obstructs the coronary arteries, blood flow to the myocardium — and oxygen along with it — decreases. Ischemia and then necrosis develop in that portion of the myocardium that's not adequately nourished. This is an acute myocardial infarction.

An AMI jeopardizes the heart's pumping mechanism. What you'll find hemodynamically includes a decrease in stroke volume, ejection fraction of the myocardium, and cardiac output. Depending on the patient, arterial pressure may be increased or decreased. Although every AMI disturbs ventricular function, the extent of the problem may not be readily evident. In some patients, life-threatening alterations can occur abruptly. So even though your patient's blood pressure may be normal, make sure you closely monitor him during this critical period.

The pain of AMI is generally substernal but may occur anywhere in the anterior chest, back, epigastrium, jaw, neck, elbow, shoulder, wrist, or forearm. The patient may describe his discomfort as a feeling of heaviness, burning, aching, choking, constriction, tightness, crushing, squeezing, or expanding. He is likely to use such expressions as, "like someone sitting on my chest," "a tight rubber band around my chest," or "feeling as if my arm would break." He may also report weakness or numbness in one or both arms.

Although severe chest pain is typical of myocardial infarction, approximately 15% of patients with AMI are asymptomatic or experience only mild discomfort, which they often don't recognize as resulting from illness. I remember Mr. Bradford, who was admitted to the CCU to rule out a diagnosis of AMI. He denied having any chest pain or arm pain. But when his nurse asked, "Is anything bothering you?" he said, "Yes, my jaw aches." His jaw pain, in fact, represented ischemic pain; serial electrocardiograms confirmed an AMI.

Other early myocardial infarction symptoms can include syncope, vertigo, nausea, vomiting, dyspnea, diaphoresis, pallor, hypotension, and hypertension. Fever is extremely rare at the onset of myocardial infarction but many times occurs in the first few days after the infarct. Remember, such fever rarely exceeds 101° F. (38.3° C.). A higher temperature (102° F., 39° C.) or persistent rise suggests complications. Notify the doctor and consider other causes.

Changes in heart sounds typical

Some patients at the onset of an AMI look normal and have normal blood pressure, pulse, and heart sounds. More usually, however, cardiac auscultation reveals characteristic changes: alterations in the intensity of heart sounds; atrial gallop (S_4); ventricular gallop (S_3); and in papillary dysfunction, an apical systolic murmur.

Patients with AMI may or may not have symptoms related to mitral regurgitation (primarily those associated with left ventricular failure and pulmonary congestion: dyspnea, rales, edema). This murmur is heard best over the mitral valve area (left side of the chest wall between the 5th and 6th intercostal spaces). It may be localized to the apex or transmitted to the left of the sternal border or to the axilla. It has a high-pitched or blowing quality but does not have to be holosystolic (per-

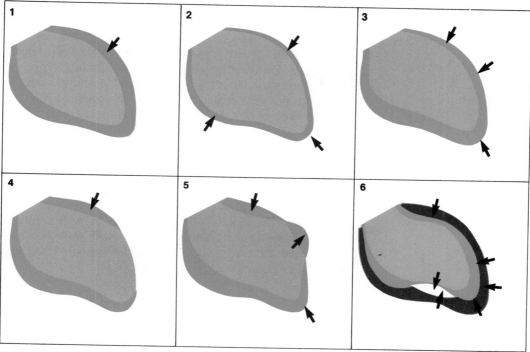

sisting throughout systole) as is the rheumatic mitral regurgitant murmur.

The doctor will locate precordial and systolic movement of the ventricle by palpating the apex, the left and right sternal borders, the suprasternal notch, and the subxiphoid. He will look for the precordial bulge (due to the paradoxical motion of the infarcted myocardium) that can accompany an AMI or tenderness, which may be caused by costochondritis.

After physical examination, patients suspected of having had a myocardial infarction always need confirming diagnostic studies. Such studies include enzyme analysis and serial EKGs. Enzyme analysis aims to detect characteristic changes in tissue levels of SGOT, LDH, and CPK (see page 88).

EKG pattern diagnostic

Q waves representing normal septal depolarization are considered normal when seen in the left precordial leads and leads aVL, L_1. The Q wave is pathologic and diagnostic for myocardial necrosis when it's wider than 0.04 second (one small

The ins and outs
1. A *normal heart* contracts in a strong uniform motion. But a heart damaged by an MI can develop left ventricular dysynergy or asynergy. 2. A *hypokinetic* contraction remains uniform but lacks force. 3. *Asyneresis* refers to a localized hypokinetic contraction. 4. *Akinesis* is the failure of a portion of the ventricular wall to contract. 5. *Dyskinesis* means a paradoxical systolic expansion or bulging of part of the ventricular wall.
6. *Asynchrony* refers to the disturbed temporal sequence of contraction.

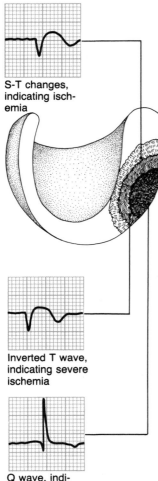

S-T changes, indicating ischemia

Inverted T wave, indicating severe ischemia

Q wave, indicating true necrosis

EKG changes with an MI
To locate an infarction, study the characteristic S-T segment and T and Q wave changes in various lead combinations. The tracings above show an elevated S-T segment — the first EKG change — and a flattened and finally inverted T wave, as well as an enlarged Q wave (indicating developing necrosis and a true infarction).

block on the graph paper) or deeper than ⅓ the height of the QRS complex. Whenever you see abnormal waves on an EKG, record their appearance, depth, and width and notify the doctor. Watch for a wide and deep Q wave with S-T segment elevation or T wave inversion — the typical infarction pattern. Expect these changes in leads oriented to the necrotic area. In leads opposite the necrotic area, look for accompanying S-T segment depression and an upright T wave (reciprocal changes). These changes represent the indirect current of injury. Look for reciprocal changes first. They're usually more obvious and will alert you to look for S-T elevation — often a more subtle change.

Infarcts can occur in the anterior, lateral, posterior, or inferior walls of the myocardium either singly or in combination (anterolateral location is common). When an AMI resolves, the S-T segment becomes less elevated; the T wave becomes less inverted and eventually upright. Often the only EKG sign of an old infarction is the pathologic Q wave.

Life-threatening complications
Anticipate and watch for complications carefully since early diagnosis and proper management may decide whether or not the patient survives.
• *Ventricular arrhythmias* are the most common and the most perilous complication. Watch for premature ventricular contractions (PVCs) that may precede ventricular tachycardia. They need immediate treatment. Ventricular arrhythmias may follow myocardial ischemia, hypotension, impaired pulmonary ventilation, hypokalemia, or drug therapy. When ventricular tachycardia is the first sign of an AMI, it forecasts a tendency to shock and congestive heart failure.
• Other arrhythmias, such as atrial tachycardia, atrial flutter or fibrillation, varying degrees of atrioventricular (AV) heart block, and sinus bradycardia, can also complicate AMI. In most instances, these arrhythmias relate to the site of the infarction and the involved arteries. For example, atrial infarction caused by right coronary artery occlusion proximal to the sinus node artery usually fosters atrial arrhythmias. Inferior infarctions frequently lead to AV block. Left anterior hemiblock and bundle-branch block may result from anterior infarction.
• *Heart failure* (mild dysfunction of the left ventricle).

Infarctions in different sites of the heart cause EKG changes. Recognizing these changes will help you assess your patient.
- An *inferior wall myocardial infarction (MI)* will show typical pattern changes — a pathologic Q wave, S-T segment elevation, and T wave inversion — in leads II, III, and aVF.
- Sometimes an inferior or posterior wall infarction will involve the lateral wall as well. *Lateral wall involvement* will cause a reduced R wave, a T wave inversion, and, in some cases, an elevation of the S-T segment in the lateral leads V_5, V_6, aVL, and L_1.
- A *posterior wall infarction* causes a tall R wave and upright T wave in V_1.

CHARACTERISTIC EKGs IN MI

- An *anterior MI* will produce a typical infarction pattern in leads I, aVL, and V_2 to V_6.
- An *anteroseptal infarction* will cause the typical pattern in leads V_1 to V_4.
- An *anterolateral infarction* will produce the typical pattern in leads I, V_5, and V_6.
- An infarction within the anterolateral surface of the left ventricle — a *high anterolateral infarction* — will produce typical changes in leads aVL, L_1, and V_6.

Change for the better
These EKG patterns gradually return to normal. Recovery after an MI can be divided into four phases:

PHASE I (acute phase): Immediately after onset or within 48 hours, leads reflecting the injured area show abnormal Q waves, an elevated S-T segment, and inverted T waves. Reciprocal changes, such as S-T depression, occur in leads reflecting the uninjured area.

PHASE II: This phase covers the gradual return of the elevated S-T segment to the baseline.

PHASE III: Most T waves return to normal or near-normal configuration.

PHASE IV (stabilized phase): An abnormal Q wave may be the only sign of infarction.

These four phases may be complete in 3 days or may take as long as 10. Remember always to interpret EKGs in light of other laboratory findings and the patient's symptoms.

COMMON ARRHYTHMIAS

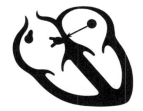

PACs

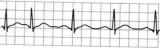

Treatment: Often none, but quinidine may be used

PAT

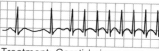

Treatment: Carotid sinus pressure, verapamil, or propranolol

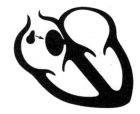

AV BLOCK — SECOND-DEGREE

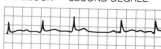

Treatment: Atropine, Isuprel, or pacemaker

AV BLOCK — THIRD-DEGREE

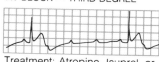

Treatment: Atropine, Isuprel, or pacemaker

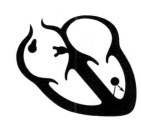

PVCs

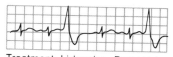

Treatment: Lidocaine, Pronestyl, or atropine, if associated with bradycardia

VENTRICULAR TACHYCARDIA

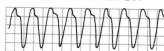

Treatment: Cardioversion (except for patients on digitalis) lidocaine, Pronestyl, or bretylium tosylate

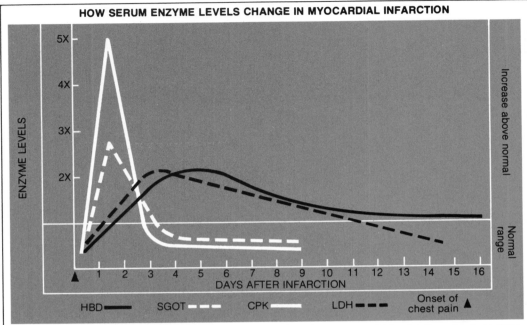

HOW SERUM ENZYME LEVELS CHANGE IN MYOCARDIAL INFARCTION

Cardiac enzymes: Critical clues

Patients suspected of having a myocardial infarction (MI) always need serial EKGs and serial enzyme studies. Enzymes are catalytic proteins that vary in concentration, depending on the tissue in which they appear. Since a damaged tissue releases enzymes into the blood, enzyme studies tell what organ is damaged and to what extent. (*Note:* Because testing methods vary from hospital to hospital, be sure to check your hospital's lab manual for normal values.)

Draw blood samples for an enzyme study very carefully, since a traumatic venipuncture can falsely elevate results. For example, red blood cells that contain LDH, HBD, and SGOT can release these enzymes in cases of hemolysis.

Look for three highly specific enzymes to help diagnose an MI:

SGOT — serum glutamic-oxaloacetic transaminase, an enzyme found mainly in the heart muscle and the liver and to some degree in skeletal muscle, kidney, and red blood cells.

LDH — lactic dehydrogenase, found in the heart, liver, kidney, brain, skeletal muscle, and erythrocytes. Since it's found in tissues outside the heart, laboratories separate LDH into five subgroups called isoenzymes. The LDH_1 and LDH_2 isoenzymes are the myocardial fraction that rises after MI. When LDH_2 is a higher value than LDH_1, the enzymes are referred to as "flipped," which is indicative of myocardial damage. Some laboratories routinely measure hydroxybutyrate dehydrogenase (HBD) as an indirect measure of LDH_1 and LDH_2.

CPK — creatine phosphoki-nase occurs in the heart, skeletal muscle, and brain, but not in red blood cells or the liver. CPK levels rise after strenuous exercise, polymyositis, muscular dystrophy, muscle injury, and MI. After skeletal muscle abnormalities and cerebral disease are ruled out, *elevated CPK is considered specific for myocardial damage.* Remember, however, intramuscular injections *alone* can elevate the CPK enzyme level. Some laboratories solve this problem by separating CPK into the following fractions or isoenzymes: CPK_1, or BB (brain tissues); CPK_2, or MB (heart muscle); and CPK_3, or MM (skeletal muscle).

When CPK is separated, *all* of the total CPK value should be CPK_3, or MM. If CPK_2, or MB, is present, it is indicative of myocardial damage, which always elevates the CPK value. A positive MB value with EKG changes is positive identification of an MI.

Watch for its signs: dyspnea, inspiratory rales at the lung bases, edema, and abnormalities in jugular venous pulsation and the carotid pulse. Mortality is 80% in patients with an AMI who develop congestive failure and pump failure (cardiogenic shock).

• *Pulmonary edema* follows left-sided heart failure. When the left side of the heart can't maintain adequate venous output, the result is increased pulmonary artery pressure and pulmonary congestion. The physical signs of pulmonary edema include dyspnea, bibasilar pulmonary rales, oliguria, and tachycardia.

• *Pump failure* occurs when MI damages the heart's ability to pump blood into the aorta in sufficient volume and pressure. Decreased cardiac output and inadequate tissue perfusion produce cardiogenic shock (in 10% to 15% of patients with AMI). You should anticipate pump failure and watch for its telltale signs: hypotension; pallor; diaphoresis; cool, clammy skin; oliguria; tachycardia; and weak, thready, rapid pulse. Such patients may also appear confused or obtunded (see also Chapter 10).

• *Pulmonary embolism* may occur in AMI patients with recurrent bouts of congestive heart failure. Suspect it when
— cyanosis is present
— heart failure doesn't respond to treatment
— unexplained pleural effusion occurs
— the patient has been on prolonged bed rest.

To prevent pulmonary embolism, encourage patients to move and exercise their legs gently and to wiggle their toes. They may benefit from antiembolism stockings. Tell such patients not to cross their legs. If they are too weak to move, give regular passive exercises to the legs, and turn them from side to side often.

• *Myocardial rupture* accounts for 10% of the AMI fatalities in the hospital. This fatal complication usually occurs within the first week after transmural infarction (involving the whole myocardial wall). Its signs include sudden worsening of the patient's condition, dyspnea, shock, and distended neck veins accompanied by pulsus paradoxus. Auscultation of the chest wall may reveal mumurs and thrills. Death can follow suddenly from cardiac tamponade (see Chapter 10). When examining a patient with cardiac tamponade, you may find electromechanical dissociation, electrical rhythmic activity

Heart-saving diet

An MI patient must watch his diet. His doctor will most likely restrict his sodium intake, so before he leaves the hospital explain the importance of avoiding the following:
• salted "snack" foods, such as potato chips and peanuts
• canned soups and vegetables
• dried fruits
• delicatessen foods, especially lox and ham
• prepared foods, such as TV dinners
• preserved meat (such as hot dogs) and luncheon meats
• cheeses of all kinds (including cottage)
• anything preserved in brine, such as olives, pickles, and sauerkraut

In addition, a patient watching calories should *avoid:*
• sugar and sweets
• high cholesterol foods
• milk, milk products, and coconut oil
• alcoholic beverages

His diet should *include* the following foods, low in sodium:

Fruits and their juices

apples	apricots
bananas	dates
grapefruit	nectarines
oranges	prunes
raisins	watermelon

Vegetables (fresh or frozen)

asparagus	beans
brussels sprouts	cabbage
cauliflower	corn
lima beans	peas
peppers	potatoes
radishes	squash

Treatment goals

Your goals for treating MI patients include relieving distress and reducing cardiac work load to allow healing and prevent extension of the infarct or complications. You can promote these goals by:

• *Relieving pain:* Usually, pain is treated with morphine, 2- to 4-mg dose, I.V. Morphine reduces anxiety and decreases cardiac work load. It also depresses respiration, reduces myocardial contractility and, by vasodilatation, decreases blood pressure and slows the heart rate. Avoid inducing hypoxia, which can induce ventricular fibrillation and cardiac arrest.

Nitroglycerin or isosorbide dinitrate also relieve pain. They redistribute blood to the ischemic area of the myocardium, increasing cardiac output and reducing myocardial work load.

• *Promoting rest:* A reduced work load helps heal the damaged myocardium and develop collateral circulation. Promote cardiac rest by enforcing bed rest, as needed (especially a challenge with an active patient who's suddenly immobilized).

Once pain has subsided, encourage patients to move their feet and legs to minimize the risk of thrombophlebitis. To check on readiness for graduated activity, watch for pain, tachycardia, or increased or decreased blood pressure before, during, and after activity. Observe for signs of pain, heart rhythm changes, or shortness of breath. If these result, the patient isn't ready to resume normal activity.

• *Preserving myocardium* vasodilators — nitrates (ointment or I.V.) — increase coronary blood flow and myocardial oxygen perfusion and maintain long-term artery dilation to meet metabolic needs. Nitrates produce more venous than arterial dilation.

(continued, opposite page)

without palpable pulses or measurable blood pressure.

• *Rupture of the intraventricular septum* accounts for 2% of all deaths within the first week after an AMI. This is due to new or old occlusions of both anterior and posterior descending arteries that supply most of the septal myocardium with blood. Watch for rapidly developing left heart failure, dyspnea, shock, and a harsh systolic murmur at the fourth left sternal border.

• *Papillary muscle rupture* is another severe complication with rapidly developing dyspnea, pulmonary edema, mitral regurgitation, and signs of decreased cardiac output.

• *Ventricular aneurysm* usually involves the left ventricle (95% of the time). Its clinical features include intractable failure, angina and arrhythmias (especially sinus tachycardia and PVCs), gallop rhythm, and a palpable systolic precordial bulge.

• *Pericarditis* occurs in 15% of patients with AMI. A pericardial friction rub appears 2 to 3 days postinfarction. It produces a pain over the precordium that is aggravated by inspiration and movement. Listen for a sound like sandpaper rubbing together. The patient who develops pericarditis usually thinks he's developing another infarction and becomes quite anxious. This pain is distinguishable from angina: it's clearly related to a change in position or breathing. It worsens during inspiration and lessens as the patient sits up in bed. The patient with pericarditis usually points to the site of pain with one finger. Anticoagulant therapy is usually contraindicated in a patient with pericarditis secondary to an AMI.

• *Dressler (postmyocardial infarction) syndrome* can occur weeks or months after an MI. The patient develops pericardial pain, pericardial friction rub, fever, left pleural effusion, arthralgia, elevated sedimentation rate, and increased serum WBCs. This syndrome, thought to be due to an antigen-antibody reaction to necrotic myocardium, needs diagnosis to distinguish it from a recurring AMI, pulmonary infarction, or congestive heart failure. Its symptoms may recur and may require steroid treatment.

Emotional problems prominent

Today, most people know what a myocardial infarction is as well as its consequences. Their natural response to it is fear and anxiety, which may endanger an already damaged heart. Stress releases catecholamines, which increase the heart rate, the force of myocardial contraction, and myocardial metabolic requirements. If the diseased heart can't cope with the greater demand for oxygen, it may develop arrhythmias, angina, heart failure, pump failure, or another MI. Clearly, patients should try to keep anxiety within tolerable limits if they're to recover.

Some patients manage their anxiety by denying their illness. Denial relieves anxiety by reducing the threat of dying and relieving the fear of the loss of good health, of being a burden, and of the loss of masculinity in the male patient. Denial is common in the first 24 to 48 hours but may persist into convalescence. When it lasts longer than 2 weeks, it can endanger the patient's welfare.

I remember one champion disbeliever, Mr. Stern. He was admitted to the CCU with an acute anterior wall myocardial infarction. His stay in the hospital was initially uneventful, and he seemed pleasantly jovial. However, after a few days we noticed that he'd talk about everything *except* his illness or its treatment. Whenever we tried to talk to him about those matters, Mr. Stern merely laughed and told jokes.

The dangerous thing about denial is that it lets patients ignore the doctor's instructions. Mr. Stern ignored his need for bed rest. He often got out of bed, unplugged his monitor, and walked to the bathroom. When reprimanded, he only laughed, saying, "I'm fine, just a little tired and short of breath. I need to walk around." His nurse explained that fatigue, shortness of breath, chest pain, and increased heart rate were caused by damage to his heart — not too much rest. She repeatedly emphasized the need for rest and finally did convince him to accept the reality of his illness.

Once denial subsides and reality sets in, depression is likely to follow. The patient who realizes how his illness will change his life is likely to feel sad, angry, or guilty. He may say things like, "Why did this happen to me? If only I had listened... quit smoking... found another job." Remember that many patients — particularly men — will need help in expressing such feelings for fear of appearing unmasculine.

Caring for a depressed patient is extremely difficult and often frustrating. Don't let your frustration lead to overprotecting or doing everything for the patient. Instead, let him know you recognize and understand his feelings, but expect him to function as he is capable. Being forced to do things for himself eases feelings of helplessness and gradually re-

Nipride I.V. dilates arterial vascular beds more than venous; decreases left ventricular filling pressure (preload); and decreases peripheral vascular resistance (afterload), causing increased cardiac output and decreased blood pressure.

In AMI patients without left ventricular dysfunction, beta-adrenergic blockers, such as propranolol (Inderal), reduce myocardial oxygen consumption by decreasing heart rate and contractility.

If you find a 10% increase in heart rate or a systolic blood pressure under 110 mm Hg in these patients, notify the doctor.

• *Combatting arrhythmias:* Lethal arrhythmias are common after AMI. Know the location of the infarct and the common arrhythmias associated with the location. Carefully monitor the patient's EKG and follow your hospital's standing orders or emergency procedures.

• *Restricting diet:* A liquid or soft diet, easily digestible foods, reduces cardiac work load.

• *Giving oxygen.* Oxygen may be given (6 to 8 L/minute), usually by nasal cannula or mask for respiratory insufficiency, dyspnea, angina, shock, or cyanosis. Patients with chronic obstructive lung disease should receive low-flow oxygen at 1 to 2 L/minute by nasal cannula.

• *Treating coronary artery thrombi:* Streptokinase dissolves acute arterial thromboemboli during transmural myocardial infarction. Initially, angiography is used to locate the blockage. Then, 3 to 6 hours after the onset of the MI, the drug is injected into the obstructed coronary artery by a long catheter inserted through a peripheral artery. It minimizes damage caused by thromboemboli by dissolving the emboli and reestablishing coronary blood flow.

stores confidence.

A special problem in men with an acute myocardial infarction is the threat to self-image and sexual adequacy. Such anxiety may appear as aggressive sexual behavior, a compensatory reaction. Instead of focusing on inappropriate behavior, try to help the patient find other ways to feel more competent and independent. Discuss the resumption of activities. Let him participate in planning his care and diet.

Your role as teacher

Throughout the patient's stay in the hospital, take primary responsibility for explaining what he can expect from the staff, what kind of information he should report, necessary procedures, monitors and other equipment, his activity, diet, fluid restriction, and so forth. Be sure to instruct the patient and his family on how to live with his illness after he goes home (see Appendices).

And don't forget to explain and prepare the patient for any moves *within* the hospital. After a few days of intensive care, most patients with AMI become conscious of their dependence on the nursing staff. They become secure in the CCU. When their condition stabilizes and they are moved to another unit, they react with great anxiety, feeling abandoned. This move can be traumatic, even dangerous, unless you prepare them for it. Don't forget their relatives, who can help support and reassure them at this time.

Remember these important points when caring for a patient with an AMI:
1. Be aware that about 15% of patients with AMI are nearly asymptomatic or have symptoms other than chest pain.
2. During auscultation, listen for characteristic AMI changes: alteration in heart sound intensity, atrial gallop (S_4), and ventricular gallop (S_3).
3. When interpreting an EKG, consider a wide and deep Q wave with S-T segment elevation, or T wave inversion indicative of an infarction.
4. Anticipate and watch for life-threatening complications, such as ventricular arrhythmias, heart failure, pulmonary edema, and pump failure.

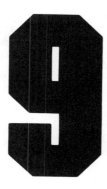

Congestive Failure
Severe cardiac impairment

BY LAUREN MARIE ISACSON, RN and
KLAUS J. SCHULZ, MD

CONGESTIVE HEART FAILURE (CHF) and its most devastating extreme, pulmonary edema, are among the most common cardiovascular problems. Their symptoms are always distressing and often potentially life-threatening. You should know how to deal with these symptoms promptly and, of course, to recognize congestive failure in all its stages. This chapter will tell you how.

Sometimes insidious

In its advanced stages, CHF is easy to recognize; as full-blown pulmonary edema, its textbook symptoms are almost impossible to miss. More often, though, chronic congestive heart failure has an insidious onset. Many patients with early congestive failure complain of having a slight cold they're unable to "shake." They may have a cough combined with some wheezing, and may have even been treated for a suspected allergy. But detailed questioning usually brings out more definitive symptoms: typically, ankle edema that appears in the evening and disappears by morning (so it may not show if you examine the patient early in the day); nocturia; and anorexia. Their anorexia may be secondary to engorgement of the liver

which may be palpable and slightly tender. A mild blow against
the right lower lateral rib cage discloses tenderness of the liver
even when it's not easily palpable or markedly enlarged. At
this stage, physical examination may reveal a few rales in the
lungs and not much else. If such patients are weight-
conscious, they usually report a puzzling, steady weight gain.

What causes these symptoms?
CHF can result from any condition that impairs cardiac function — most commonly arteriosclerotic heart disease,
myocardial infarction, hypertension, rheumatic valvular disease, or congenital heart anomalies. In most patients with
these diseases, the left ventricle becomes damaged and eventually fails. Blood backs up in the left atrium and the pulmonary capillary bed. The lungs act as a sponge and take up some
of this extra fluid. Eventually they, too, become overloaded
and symptoms of pulmonary edema begin.

Left-sided failure is the kind most likely after myocardial
infarction. Its symptoms reflect: increased pulmonary congestion and pressure, and decreased blood flow to all tissues
and organs. In such patients, expect to see: dyspnea on exertion or at rest, tachypnea, orthopnea, paroxysmal nocturnal
dyspnea, cough, pulmonary rales, (which may be audible
without a stethoscope), fatigue, mental confusion, sodium and
water retention, and decreased tolerance to physical activity.

Right-sided failure often follows left-sided failure because
the right side must then pump against the increased resistance
in the pulmonary system. Patients with right-sided failure typically develop dependent edema, coolness of the extremities,
hepatomegaly, occasional abdominal pain, ascites, neck-vein
distention, and increased venous pressure. They usually show
a positive hepatojugular reflux. The tell-tale sign is neck-vein
distention when the patient is upright. Neck veins may show
abnormal pulsations, look distended, and feel rigid — all signs
of high venous pressure.

In many elderly people, who tend to have both arteriosclerosis and some degenerative changes due to age, both
ventricles begin to fail at the same time. Both chambers falter
in their capacity to pump blood into the circulation; consequently, symptoms of left and right ventricular failure develop simultaneously. In such patients, the symptoms may
not, at first, clearly suggest CHF.

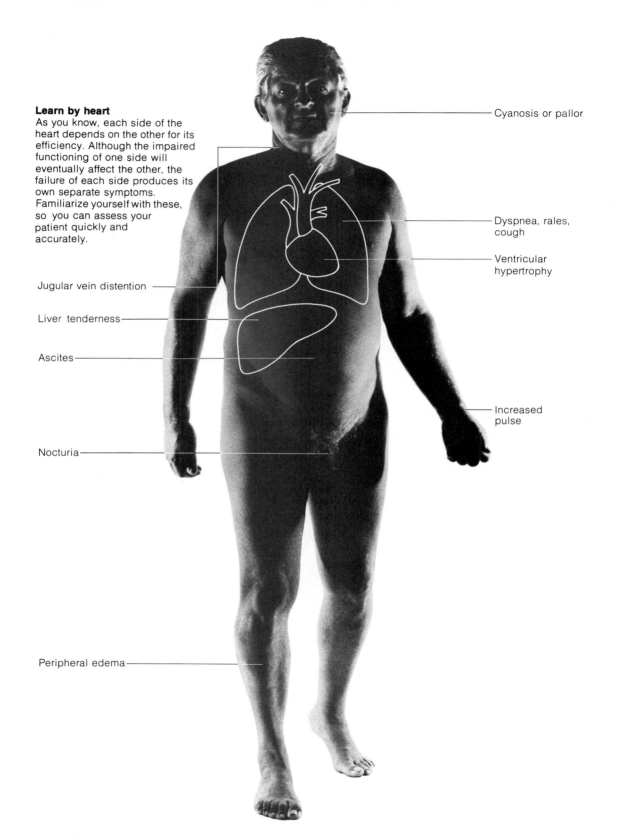

Learn by heart
As you know, each side of the heart depends on the other for its efficiency. Although the impaired functioning of one side will eventually affect the other, the failure of each side produces its own separate symptoms. Familiarize yourself with these, so you can assess your patient quickly and accurately.

Cyanosis or pallor

Dyspnea, rales, cough

Ventricular hypertrophy

Jugular vein distention

Liver tenderness

Ascites

Increased pulse

Nocturia

Peripheral edema

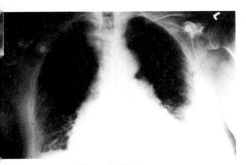

Pleural effusion
Roughly one third of patients with congestive heart failure develop pleural effusion — a collection of fluid in the pleural lining of the lungs. How does this happen? In patients with CHF, high venous pressure obstructs lymphatic absorption of the fluid that lubricates the pleura and causes this fluid to accumulate.

You can't easily see a pleural effusion on an X-ray unless more than 300 ml of fluid have accumulated; then you may see some blunting of the costophrenic angle. But you should be able to notice the reduction or absence of breath sounds at the base of the lung where the fluid collects. If it accumulates quickly, it may actually shift the mediastinum to one side, displacing the lungs and causing dyspnea. A patient in this situation may have an irregular breathing pattern.

Treatment aims to correct the CHF. Still, good pulmonary hygiene is important. Tell the patient to avoid lying on the side of the effusion to allow lung expansion and prevent atelectasis. If he's short of breath, he'll feel better in upright or semi-Fowler's position. Aspiration by thoracentesis may be needed.

Mrs. Bradford's case illustrates such insidious onset: Mrs. Bradford was quite upset when she came to her doctor's office. She had always been an active, healthy woman and had enjoyed raising her children, cooking the extravagant meals her family loved, and successfully running a rooming house. At age 62, she saw no reason to slow down. But for the last 6 months, she'd been plagued by a persistent "cold." She tired easily, was often short of breath, and from time to time had an annoying cough, especially at night. Lately, she had to use three pillows under her head to get any rest. She'd been treated for allergies, but nothing seemed to help.

Mrs. Bradford's physical examination quickly identified the source of her problems: Auscultation and percussion revealed left ventricular enlargement and a systolic murmur. Inspection revealed other signs of right heart failure: jugular vein distention, an enlarged liver, positive hepatojugular reflux, and marked peripheral edema. An EKG showed a rapid heart rate (120 BPM) and ventricular hypertrophy (a possible clue to etiology). Chest X-rays confirmed congestive heart failure: They showed pulmonary vascular congestion and some pleural effusion (see insert).

The cause of Mrs. Bradford's congestive heart failure was thought to be arteriosclerotic hypertensive disease. This was confirmed via hypertensive arteriosclerotic changes on the eye grounds exam and in echocardiography, her own history, and her family history. Another supporting fact: At 168 pounds, she was markedly overweight for her short (5 foot) stature. Mrs. Bradford was successfully treated with digitalis, a diuretic, and a 1500-calorie, low-sodium diet.

All of this happened 14 years ago. Since then Mrs. Bradford has had regular checkups. At 76, she still enjoys good health for a woman of her age. She weighs 138 pounds. Her X-ray shows normal heart size, and her lungs are clear. Her heart rate has slowed to a normal 68, and she has no more dyspnea or ankle edema. Most important to Mrs. Bradford, she can enjoy a good night's rest and has the vitality for a normal life.

Mrs. Bradford wisely sought medical help at an early stage of CHF. Patients who delay develop more dramatic signs: more rales, more distention of the neck veins, dullness over the lower chest area due to pleural effusion, markedly enlarged liver, and pitting ankle edema. (Bedridden patients develop edema over the sacrum.)

Treatment commonplace

In all stages of CHF, treatment is relatively similar. It always includes:

- diuresis via diuretics
- semirecumbent position for a day or two to drain edema and decrease cardiac work load
- prevention of electrolyte imbalance
- digitalis to augment myocardial contractility
- nitrates to reduce preload
- vasodilators (Nipride, Apresoline, Minipress) to increase cardiac output by reducing the impedance to ventricular outflow (afterload)
- converting enzyme inhibitor (captopril) to prevent production of angiotensin II from angiotensin I, thereby reducing preload and afterload.

If the patient has not taken digitalis before, a digitalizing dose is given the first day followed by maintenance doses. (So be sure to take an accurate drug history.)

In difficult cases, standard drug treatment may seem ineffective, and various drugs and dosages may need to be tried. In such cases, weigh the patient daily to assess fluid status. Monitor fluid intake, urine output, and vital signs. Auscultate the heart and lungs frequently for abnormal sounds (S_3 and rales). Notify the doctor of any change.

Throughout treatment, your nursing observations and care are crucial. Your observations begin at admission with baseline assessment of the patient's physical and mental status. This assessment should always include the patient's weight and vital signs: temperature, pulse, respirations, and blood pressure. Observe the patient's appearance and take a thorough nursing history. Usually the complete history has to wait, since such patients are in great distress when first hospitalized. But the physical appearance, vital signs, and mental state are a mandatory baseline for measuring the effects of treatment.

Three stages of pulmonary edema

In its severest form, CHF causes pulmonary edema — an extreme emergency. Pulmonary edema almost always has its source in left ventricular failure that increases pressure in the pulmonary vascular bed and forces fluid and solutes from the intravascular compartment into the interstitium of the lungs (see insert on the following page).

A closer look at the lungs

The lungs consist of three different anatomical entities which interconnect and influence each other. The first anatomical structure, the network of airways, consists of the trachea, major bronchi, small bronchial tubules, and alveoli. The second, or circulatory network, includes the pulmonary arteries, veins, arterioles, venules, and the capillary bed. These two networks are imbedded in the third, called the interstitium or interstitial space, which is composed of connective tissue.

The alveolar membranes and the pulmonary capillary membranes share a common basement membrane which facilitates the exchange of oxygen and carbon dioxide with the blood. The small alveolar vessels are chiefly involved in the function of gas exchange, while the extra-alveolar vessels and the lymphatics both help regulate fluid and solute movement within the interstitium. If the vascular compartment overloads with fluids, lymphatics ordinarily can drain away the excess.

Normally, the pressure in the pulmonary vascular bed is higher than in the surrounding interstitium. This pressure difference facilitates the movement of fluids out of the capillaries. However, solutes such as plasma proteins within capillaries exert serum colloid osmotic pressure which prevents too much fluid and electrolytes from leaving the vascular bed. Pulmonary edema can easily arise when this balance is disturbed.

1. *Interstitial stage.* Patients in this stage become short of breath with any exercise. They have difficulty climbing stairs. They can't sleep in a supine position because of dyspnea and spend whole nights sitting upright in a chair (orthopnea). They try to compensate by hyperventilating and so their PCO_2 falls while their PO_2 remains near or slightly below normal. They may complain of restlessness and a feeling of anxiety. During physical assessment of patients in this stage, you're likely to pick up an abnormal third heart sound, the diastolic gallop.

As the interstitium continues to swell with fluids, the lymphatic system can no longer handle the fluid overload. Fluid floods into the peripheral alveoli, further blocking adequate gas exchange. Now the patient's respiratory rate climbs and his auxiliary respiratory muscles begin to work. The increased respiratory effort uses up large amounts of oxygen, deepening the oxygen debt.

2. *Alveolar stage.* At this stage, both PO_2 and PCO_2 drop considerably below normal. As the PCO_2 falls, the pH rises. Hyperventilation blows off too much CO_2 and causes respiratory alkalosis. These rapid, labored respirations increase venous return to the heart, adding more venous blood to an already overloaded pulmonary capillary bed. Hypoxia increases and, in turn, triggers the release of catecholamines to stimulate cardiac action.

At this stage, an examiner can easily hear characteristic crepitant rales (bubbles of edema fluid mixed with surfactant, a lipid protein that coats the walls of the alveoli and keeps them from collapsing). When air goes through these fluid-filled alveoli, it makes this characteristic sound.

3. *Bronchial stage.* In the third stage, the small bronchioles begin to retain fluid. Now the bubbles are larger, and the sounds they make are not fine crepitant rales but coarse bubbling sounds. The bronchial tree tends to become spastic, causing the patient to wheeze. Such wheezing may cause the examiner to suspect asthma — hence this condition is sometimes called cardiac asthma.

As the bronchial tree fills with fluid, the patient's condition deteriorates. His arterial blood gas (ABG) studies show a sharp drop in PO_2. Tissues respond to the dwindling oxygen supply by resorting to anaerobic metabolism. This pours large quantities of lactic acid into the bloodstream, creating metabolic acidosis. The patient may begin wheezing and

MANAGING A PATIENT WITH PULMONARY EDEMA		
STAGES	SYMPTOMS	NURSING RESPONSIBILITIES
INITIAL	• Persistent cough — patient feels "like a cold is coming on" • Slight dyspnea/orthopnea • Exercise intolerance • Restlessness • Anxiety • Crepitant rales may be heard over the dependent portion of the lungs • Diastolic gallop	• Check color and amount of expectoration. • Position patient for comfort. • Auscultate chest for rales and third heart sound. • Medicate as ordered. • Monitor apical and radial pulses for rate and rhythm. • Assist patient with all needs to conserve strength. • Provide emotional support (through all stages) for patient and family.
ADVANCED	• Acute shortness of breath • Respirations — rapid, noisy (audible wheeze, rales) • Cough more intense and productive of frothy, blood-tinged sputum • Cyanosis • Diaphoresis — skin cold and clammy • Tachycardia — arrhythmias • Hypotension	• Institute emergency measures: — Give oxygen — preferably by high concentration mask or IPPB. — Insert I.V. if not already done. — Aspirate nasopharynx p.r.n. — Give digitalis and morphine, as ordered. — Give potent diuretics (e.g., furosemide [Lasix] or ethacrynic acid [Edecrin]), as ordered. — Insert Foley catheter. — Calculate intake and output exactly. — Draw ABGs. — Attach cardiac monitor leads and observe EKG. — Prepare for phlebotomy, if necessary. — Have resuscitation equipment available.
ACUTE	• Decreased level of consciousness • Ventricular arrhythmias • Shock • Diminished breath sounds	• Give emotional support to patient and family. • Be prepared for cardioversion of tachyarrhythmias. • Assist with intubation and mechanical ventilation. • Resuscitate if necessary.

cough up blood-tinged sputum. *His PCO_2 may start to level off, but don't mistake this for an improvement. It's a sign of incipient respiratory failure.*

In this final stage, pulmonary edema leaves the patient severely hypoxic and exhausted from nearly fruitless respiratory efforts. His PCO_2 rises markedly, and the combined sequelae of respiratory and metabolic acidosis put him in a precarious condition. Without immediate treatment, the patient will die. Such treatment always includes administration of diuretics and morphine, and adequate oxygenation (see chart above).

Mr. Stevens' case illustrates the details of such treatment. Less than 2 hours after calmly sitting down to watch his favorite television show, Mr. Stevens was in our emergency department...in acute distress. His skin felt cold and clammy, he had an elevated blood pressure, and he was cyanotic. His

Non-cardiac causes of P.E.
Conditions other than heart failure can cause pulmonary edema, such as:
• Toxins from infections or inhalants, and vasoactive substances, such as histamines, that increase capillary permeability, allow excess fluids into the lungs;
• Renal and hepatic diseases, and some nutritional disturbances that decrease serum colloid osmotic pressure, cause fluids to accumulate in the pulmonary interstitium;
• Diseases, such as Hodgkin's, that block normal lymphatic drainage, permit fluids to accumulate.

respirations sounded bubbly, with moist rales over both lungs. He had frothy, blood-tinged secretions in the corners of his mouth.

Mr. Stevens was in the final stage of respiratory failure from fulminating pulmonary edema. We quickly elevated his head, cleared his airway, then administered oxygen. He looked anxious and frightened, and became even more so as we hovered over him. A patient who fears that any moment he may stop breathing compounds his difficulties by expending more oxygen and producing more carbon dioxide than he would if he were calmer. So in low, confident tones, we continually explained what we were doing — why we were giving him oxygen, why we were starting an I.V., why we were repeatedly taking vital signs.

If a patient can cough and expectorate, he may be able to clear his airway. If he can't he'll need to be suctioned, as did Mr. Stevens. Once we'd made certain of an open airway and had drawn blood for an arterial blood gas analysis, we started him on high-concentration oxygen by mask. (The commonly used nasal cannula doesn't deliver enough oxygen to meet the needs of a patient with pulmonary edema.)

Mr. Stevens' initial ABG readings clearly showed that he was unable to maintain adequate ventilation on his own. With a pH of 7.0, a PCO_2 of 84, and a PO_2 of 64, he needed to be intubated immediately if we were to save his life. We quickly inserted an endotracheal tube and began ventilating him on an MA-1 respirator, FIO_2 100%. (Remember that oxygen must be administered in precisely prescribed doses or you risk over-oxygenating your patient. Avoid over-oxygenation by checking ABGs frequently and adjusting the ventilator accordingly. (see insert, *Checklist for Patients Receiving Oxygen*).

Mr. Stevens' respiratory acidosis was corrected quickly. His pH rose to 7.44 and his PCO_2 dropped to 32. However, despite the 100% oxygen, his PO_2 increased only to 96, meaning that much of his cardiac output was still being shunted past fluid-filled alveoli.

Drug regimen
To remove the excess alveolar fluid, we started I.V. diuretics with 40 mg of furosemide (Lasix). To keep track of his intake and output, we inserted a Foley catheter. Along with the diuretic, we gave Mr. Stevens an initial intravenous dose of

A CHECKLIST FOR PATIENTS RECEIVING OXYGEN				
METHOD OF OXYGEN DELIVERY	FLOW RATE	PERCENTAGE OF OXYGEN DELIVERY (FIO₂)	PURPOSE OF TREATMENT	CAUTIONS
Nasal cannula	2-6 L/min	Up to 55%	Corrects hypoxia; decreases breathing efforts; lessens the work load of the heart.	Dries mucous membranes of nose and throat. Keep nasal passages clean.
Medium concentration mask	8-10 L/min (Never less than 5 L/min)	40%-70%	Same as above.	Fearing suffocation patients tolerate mask poorly. Keep face dry under mask to prevent irritation.
High concentration (non-rebreathing bag) mask	Sufficient to keep bag inflated. 6-10 L/min	60%-95%	Same as above.	Never allow bag to collapse completely during inspiration. Maintain a tight seal.
IPPB (Intermittent Positive Pressure Breathing)	Preset rate and volume	40%-80%	Decreases breathing efforts; improves patient's coughing mechanism; delivers bronchodilators; decreases venous return to heart; helps expand the lungs.	Discontinue treatment if hemoptysis occurs. Use temporarily in pulmonary edema. Contraindicated in pneumothorax without chest tube. Watch patient for tachycardia and dyspnea.
CMV (Continuous Mechanical Ventilation) Assist	Preset rate and volume	21%-100% as required	Augments patient's own ventilatory cycle; a determined amount of gas and oxygen is inspired.	Check ABGs frequently. Reassure and sedate patient as needed.
CMV (Continuous Mechanical Ventilation) Controlled	Preset rate and volume	21%-100% as required	Assumes total work of breathing.	Provide means for communication. Check settings.
CPAP (Continuous Positive Airway Pressure) Used on patient breathing spontaneously	Set as determined by patient's ABGs, age, and type of equipment used		Alleviates respiratory distress syndrome.	Check for decreasing cardiac output. Watch for pneumothorax.
PEEP (Positive End Expiratory Pressure) Used in intubated patients with suitable respirator or Ambu bag with PEEP valve	Same as above		Increases the lungs' functional residual capacity to its normal level (improves lung compliance); improves oxygenation without use of dangerously high oxygen concentration.	Hypotension may occur. Watch for signs of pneumothorax.

morphine, 4 mg, to reduce anxiety, and nitroglycerin ointment (Nitrol). Nitroglycerin causes a pooling of venous blood that decreases the heart's work load by lowering ventricular diastolic pressure and reducing the stretching of myocardial fibers.

Fortunately, Mr. Stevens recovered sufficiently with repeated doses of diuretics and nitroglycerin ointment. After 24 hours, he no longer needed ventilatory assistance. If he had not responded, other treatments could have been added. Aminophylline may help dilate bronchi and increase cardiac output. (But give this drug slowly to prevent a sudden — possibly fatal — drop in blood pressure.) Sodium bicarbonate may also be ordered for severe metabolic acidosis.

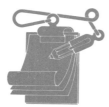

Remember these important points when assessing for and coping with CHF:
1. Look for early symptoms, such as wheezing, coughing, ankle edema at night, nocturia, and anorexia.
2. Know that left-sided failure is most common after an MI, and that right-sided failure often follows left-sided failure.
3. As ordered, administer diuretics to promote diuresis and digitalis to augment myocardial contractility; place patient in a semirecumbent position to drain edema and decrease cardiac work load; and closely monitor electrolytes to prevent imbalance.
4. Reassure a patient who's responding to treatment that he can resume a normal life by continuing therapy with digitalis and diuretics under his doctor's supervision.
5. Watch for signs of pulmonary edema, a life-threatening CHF complication: cough, exercise intolerance, restlessness, anxiety, cyanosis, hypotension, and tachycardia.

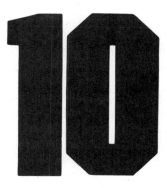

Cardiac Complications
Often catastrophic

BY SALLY A. BOWERS, RN

ONCE A PATIENT WITH severe cardiac dysfunction has been admitted to a coronary care unit, his chances of survival are reasonably good — unless he develops certain complications. To detect these complications before they become catastrophic, you must know: what these complications are; what you can do to prevent them; how to detect them in their earliest, most treatable stages; and what the appropriate treatment is so you can give it promptly.

The major complications are these: cardiogenic shock, ventricular aneurysm, and cardiac tamponade.

Cardiogenic shock — most perilous
Cardiogenic shock is now the major complication leading to death in patients with myocardial infarction. Ten to 15% of patients with MI develop cardiogenic shock; their mortality rate is 85% or greater.

How to recognize it? Usually, the patient in cardiogenic shock has cold, clammy skin and a systolic blood pressure below 80 mm Hg. But don't be fooled by an initially normal blood pressure. Hypertensive patients may drop their blood pressure 20 to 30 mm Hg and still have a systolic pressure over

The Swan-Ganz catheter

A reliable index of left ventricular function is the left-ventricular end-diastolic pressure (LVEDP), obtained with a Swan-Ganz catheter (see page 105). When pumping is insufficient, left ventricular blood volume and then the LVEDP, left atrial pressure (LAP), pulmonary arterial pressure (PAP), and pulmonary wedge pressures (PWP) can all rise. The normal pressures? LVEDP, 12 mm Hg or less; PAP, 25/10 mm Hg; and PWP, 4 to 12 mm Hg. In cardiogenic shock, you're likely to see a PWP greater than 15 mm Hg because of left ventricular failure.

Closely monitor the EKG for ventricular irritability while the doctor inserts the Swan-Ganz. Have lidocaine and a defibrillator handy. Once the catheter is in place, monitor the PAP continuously. Keep the line patent with a pressurized, heparinized flush solution.

If you get a poor pressure tracing, check to make sure all connections are tight, stopcocks are turned in the right direction, the catheter hasn't kinked, there are no air bubbles in the tubing or connections, and the balloon is deflated. A dampened tracing may indicate that the catheter is clotting or may not be in the correct position. Try to aspirate the clot and flush the catheter, but not unless the clot can be withdrawn or the catheter can be pulled back 5 cm. Avoid using the catheter to draw blood samples because this increases the chance of clotting within the catheter.

Use the PA line for pressure readings only, not as another I.V. line for medications. To avoid the need to reposition the catheter, make sure it's firmly secured to the patient's chest so it won't be pulled out of place inadvertently.

90. Other symptoms include pallor, cyanosis, mental confusion or lethargy, and urine output less than 20 ml/hour.

Watch for subtle changes in the patient's sensorium — they may be your first clue to impending shock. You'd expect a patient who has suffered a heart attack to be concerned and anxious. But *undue* restlessness and confusion should make you suspect poor cerebral vascular perfusion from a falling cardiac output. A patient in this situation can quickly deteriorate into coma.

Another result of decreased cardiac output is overall hypoxemia. Consequently, the arterial blood gas determinations in patients with cardiogenic shock show a markedly depressed PO_2. This hypoxemia can cause metabolic (lactic) acidosis and low pH. You must correct such acidosis promptly, since it further weakens myocardial function and may make the heart refractory to certain drugs, particularly the vasopressors.

Systolic blood pressure usually falls before diastolic, so you may notice a narrowing pulse pressure. If the patient is hypertensive, consider a drop to 100 mm Hg, or to 40 mm Hg below baseline level, definite hypotension. When such hypotension accompanies oliguria (urine output below 20 ml/hour) and other signs of diminished cardiac output (cyanosis and confusion), cardiogenic shock is probably present. Urine output falls because inadequate kidney perfusion activates the renin-angiotensin system to release angiotensin, an active vasopressor. At the same time, increased aldosterone stimulates the kidney to retain sodium and water.

Once you're sure hypotension is present, rule out possible causes of precipitous fall in blood pressure: pain, excessive analgesia, excessive diuresis, hypoxemia, arrhythmias, trinitrates, and antihypertensive drugs. Remember that tachycardia and bradycardia can cause a shock-like syndrome, but its symptoms are reversible once the arrhythmia is corrected. So, if the patient has tachycardia or bradycardia, antiarrhythmic treatment alone may boost cardiac output.

Rule out extracardiac causes

Quickly evaluate possible extracardiac causes for shock so that appropriate treatment can begin. For example, hypoxia from extracardiac (respiratory) causes may impair cardiac function; in such cases, improving respiration reverses shock.

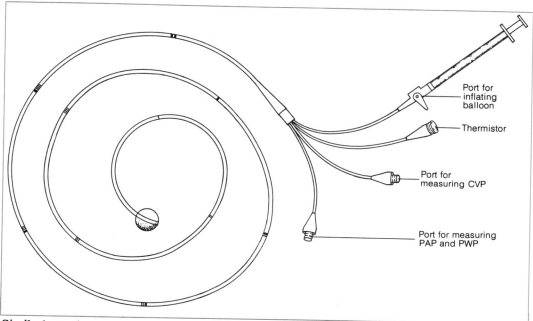

Port for
inflating
balloon

Thermistor

Port for
measuring CVP

Port for measuring
PAP and PWP

Similarly, pain may cause a vasovagal response mimicking shock; effective analgesia will counteract it. Morphine and myocardial antiarrhythmic drugs can decrease cardiac output and blood pressure. So, evaluate their effects carefully as another possible cause of shock. If shock persists after all these factors have been eliminated or treated, evaluate central venous pressure (CVP), or, more reliably, the left ventricular end-diastolic pressure (LVEDP) (see page 104). If the pulmonary arterial pressure is low or normal, begin treatment to expand blood volume.

Four ways to measure
Doctors use this Swan-Ganz Thermodilution catheter — a quadruple-lumen catheter inserted into the right heart — to measure cardiac output, CVP, pulmonary artery pressure, and pulmonary wedge pressure. One port contains a thermistor tip to which the cardiac output monitor is connected.

Treatment

Treatment of cardiogenic shock aims to increase blood pressure and coronary artery perfusion and thereby improve cardiac function. Specifically, such treatment should increase cardiac output and preserve ischemic myocardium by decreasing preload (related to LVEDP), afterload (stress in the ventricular wall during muscle shortening), and myocardial oxygen consumption. Treatment usually begins with intravenous infusions to expand blood volume, if hypovolemia is present. Hypovolemia can result from many things such as

Nursing actions for IABP problems

Thrombus formation due to blood cells clumping around balloon or decreased blood flow in affected limb: Check perfusion in extremities; watch for CVA; administer I.V. heparin carefully as ordered; check clotting times daily.

Hemorrhage or thrombocytopenia due to platelet destruction by IABP and anticoagulant therapy: Check dressings over arterial lines, Swan-Ganz, pacemaker, and IABP insertion site for bleeding qlh; order daily CBC and clotting studies (platelet count will decrease slightly in patient on heparin and IABP); administer packed cells and platelets as ordered.

Volume depletion and anemia due to too many blood samples: Tell doctor how much blood work is being done.

Lower perfusion to renal arteries and left arm due to balloon displacement: Check urine volume and specific gravity qlh; check balloon position on X-ray; check perfusion to extremities.

IABP malfunction due to poor triggering from arrhythmias: Treat

(continued, opposite page)

excessive diuresis, rigid fluid restriction, emesis from digitalis toxicity, hemorrhages and subcutaneous hematomas (after anticoagulants), or prolonged use of vasopressors.

If the PA wedge pressure is less than 15 mm Hg, you can try a fluid challenge — usually with rapid infusion of salt-poor albumin (100 ml in 10 to 15 minutes). But crystalline solutions, such as saline or dextrose in water, may also be used. In either case, this therapy is hazardous, so monitor it carefully. Record baseline pressures before the infusion starts; measure them again in the middle and at the end of the infusion. Make sure I.V. lines are patent and avoid interstitial infiltration. Consider fluid infusion helpful if blood pressure and urine output improve without a rapid rise in pulmonary wedge pressure. However, if you find pulmonary rales and congestion, discontinue the infusion immediately. If arterial pressure does not improve after the infusion (that is, systolic remains below 90 mm Hg) and if urine output remains below 20 ml/hour, the doctor will add drug treatment to improve cardiac function.

Cardiac drugs

Such treatment might include intravenous dopamine, which in small doses may not significantly increase myocardial oxygen demands. Dopamine dilates all vascular beds, increases mesenteric and renal blood flow, and improves cardiac output by decreasing afterload and preload.

What's the dosage? Usually, an ampul of dopamine (5 ml/ 200 mg) is diluted in 250 to 500 ml of a dextrose or saline solution. It's infused at a rate of 5 to 30 mcg/kg/minute (or maximum 50 mcg/kg/minute). Whenever possible, infuse dopamine into a large vein to avoid extravasation with necrosis and sloughing of surrounding tissue. Dopamine is best given with an infusion pump or microdrip regulator to avoid an inadvertent bolus and gross fluctuations in blood pressure.

During dopamine infusion, monitor for sinus tachycardia or atrial or ventricular arrhythmias. Such arrhythmias may occur at the beginning of dopamine infusion, but usually subside after 15 to 20 minutes. If they persist (or if blood pressure does not improve), dopamine may have to be discontinued and another drug substituted. Norepinephine is sometimes used. It does increase the rate and force of myocardial contraction, but has the disadvantage of increasing oxygen demand. Most doctors avoid giving isoproterenol because it shunts cardiac output to nonvital areas (skin and skeletal muscle). And it decreases oxygen supply to the myocardium by lowering diastolic perfusion pressure.

When a vasopressor can maintain blood pressure above 90 to 100 mm Hg, concomitant use of a vasodilator (nitroprusside, Nipride) further improves cardiac output by reducing afterload (as it lowers aortic systolic pressure). Far more potent and shorter acting than the nitrates, nitroprusside relaxes both arteries and veins. It takes effect very rapidly (within minutes) and can cause cyanide toxicity. So check serum thiocyanate levels every 72 hours and monitor carefully for signs of thiocyanate toxicity as well as tachycardia, ventricular arrhythmias, or falling blood pressure. If blood pressure drops below 80 mm Hg or any of these signs occur, stop the infusion. Nitroprusside is light-sensitive, so cover the solution bag and infusion lines with nontransparent paper or foil. Discard any solution after 24 hours since the drug loses potency after that time.

Take samples for blood-gas determinations every 4 hours to see that the PO_2 level stays higher than 75 mm Hg. The patient may need oxygen therapy or intubation and mechanical ventilation for adequate oxygen exchange. He may also need sodium bicarbonate to correct metabolic acidosis.

The patient will need circulatory assist next if, after treatment, cardiac output is less than 2 L/minute; if systolic pressure is less than 80 mm Hg (or 100 mm Hg in a previously hypertensive patient); or if urinary output is less than 20 ml/hour.

Help for the failing heart

The intraaortic balloon pump (IABP) is commonly used to increase coronary perfusion and assist the failing heart by decreasing its work load. It can sometimes save lives of patients with cardiogenic shock.

The balloon catheter is a thin-walled pumping chamber. It is introduced into one of the femoral arteries (whichever one has the stronger pulse) and passed up the aorta into a position just distal to the left subclavian artery. Inflation of the balloon is triggered by the patient's own EKG. It inflates during ventricular diastole (displacing blood proximally and increasing blood flow to the coronary arteries). It deflates before systole, before the aortic valve opens, allowing the ventricle to

arrhythmias as ordered; for sinus tachycardia (110 BPM), use a 2:1 trigger; for supraventricular tachycardia, try drugs or assist with cardioversion; use external pacing for bradycardia or to override accelerated rhythm.

Diastolic augmentation below optimum: To determine reason for reduced augmentation, check arterial line patency, kinks in IABP catheter, bend in affected limb, need to refill balloon with carbon dioxide or helium, position of balloon, and timing adjustments.

Timing below optimum due to early inflation or late deflation: Readjust timing according to manufacturer's guidelines or notify the person responsible for the balloon pump adjustments.

Restricted mobility due to many lines and catheters: Use passive and active exercises for limbs, as tolerated; turn and position patient, but don't elevate his head more than 30° because of balloon location; avoid sharp flexion of the leg.

Sleep deprivation, disorientation, or denial in conscious patient: Explain equipment and procedures carefully; plan continuity of care, using same staff members each shift, if possible; use medications to promote relaxation and emotional stability, if condition permits.

Always keep an IABP machine set on automatic alarm.

When not to wean

Discontinue weaning a patient from an intra-aortic balloon pump if any of the following physical signs develop:
- Hypotension
- Increased pulmonary wedge pressure (PWP)
- Decreased urine output
- Clouding sensorium
- Angina
- S-T or T wave changes indicating ischemia
- Arrhythmias (PVCs) or change in heart rate.

contract against lower pressure and decreasing the afterload.

A cardiovascular surgeon usually inserts the balloon catheter at bedside and confirms its position on chest film. The balloon should be distal to the left subclavian artery in the thoracic aorta. Change the dressings over the balloon insertion site daily, using sterile technique. And watch for signs of infection.

Monitor constantly for hemodynamic changes. In case of ventricular fibrillation or cardiac arrest, turn the balloon pump off during external cardiac massage to prevent injury to the heart (see page 113). It's possible to coordinate chest compression with automatic balloon inflation and deflation, but the precise timing needed is difficult to maintain in an emergency situation.

Consider the response to IABP satisfactory if....
- blood pressure rises
- urinary output increases
- the patient is alert
- CVP and pulmonary arterial wedge pressures are normal
- vasopressors are no longer needed.

The patient can then be weaned from the balloon. How? By gradually decreasing the volume of gas inflating the balloon, or by decreasing the ratio at which the balloon inflates (1:2 to 1:6).

But if there's been no circulatory improvement (see insert above), the patient may be continued on the balloon (as long as several weeks) or evaluated for surgery. For example, arteriography can be done with the balloon in place to check the extent of infarction and coronary artery occlusion. Depending on the findings, the patient may need coronary bypass or resection of the ventricular wall (infarctectomy). Unfortunately, most patients in cardiogenic shock are too sick to make surgery feasible.

Mr. Levinthal's case illustrates the complexities of treating cardiogenic shock.

Mr. Levinthal, a 58-year-old foreman, was hospitalized with acute inferior wall myocardial infarction. He had a history of hypertension and an earlier myocardial infarction. At admission, his blood pressure was 130/85; pulse 110, sinus; respirations 34. He had severe chest pain and pulmonary edema. We quickly established an I.V. with 5% dextrose in water and gave nasal oxygen at 4L/min. We gave morphine sulphate, 4 mg, and furosemide (Lasix), 40 mg, (both intravenously), and

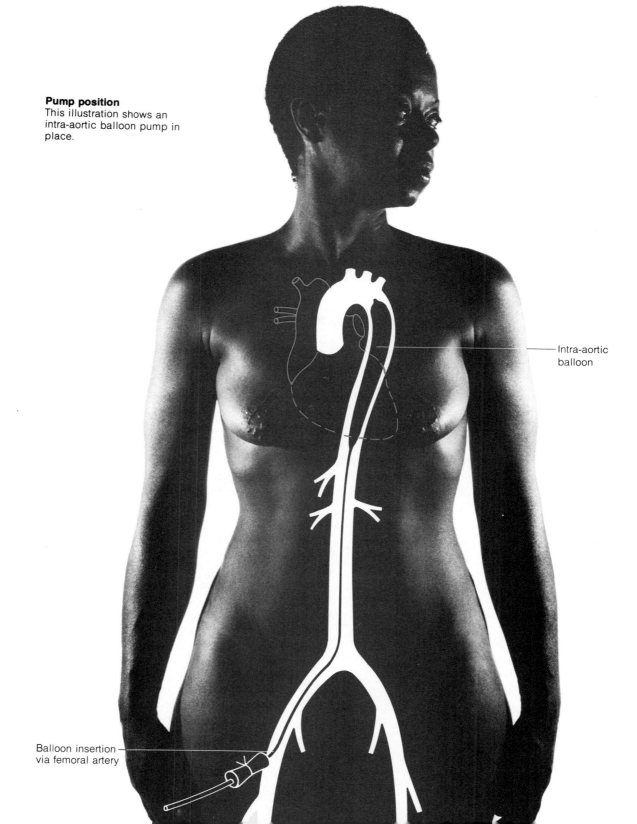

Pump position
This illustration shows an intra-aortic balloon pump in place.

Intra-aortic balloon

Balloon insertion via femoral artery

applied rotating tourniquets. We inserted a urinary catheter, which drained 200 ml of urine. Over the next several hours, Mr. Levinthal's BP fell to 80/50; his pulse rate rose to 120; his respirations to 36. He became increasingly lethargic; the doctor suspected cardiogenic shock. Dopamine (Intropin) was added to 5% dextrose in water and an infusion was begun.

At this point, Mr. Levinthal was semiconscious and profoundly cyanotic. His blood pressure was 100/70 mm Hg; PCO_2, 32 mm Hg; PO_2, 56 mm Hg; and pH, 7.28. An EKG showed sinus tachycardia with occasional unifocal PVCs. For the previous 2 hours, his urine output had been only 10 ml. The doctor decided to intubate and placed Mr. Levinthal on a ventilator with FIO_2 at 60%. On the ventilator, Mr. Levinthal's PO_2 rose to 78 mm Hg; PCO_2 was 36 mm Hg; and pH, 7.31. He was given an ampul (50 ml-44 mEq) of sodium bicarbonate, and his FIO_2 was raised to 70%. He still remained barely conscious.

A Swan-Ganz catheter was inserted. His PA mean pressure was 30 mm Hg; cardiac output was 2.9 L/minute. An intraarterial catheter was inserted in his left radial artery, and preparations made for insertion of an IABP. The dopamine infusion was increased to the rate of 20 mcg/kg/minute. Blood pressure remained low at around 95/70. Urine output improved slightly in the next hour to 20 ml/hour.

A 45-ml balloon catheter was inserted through the left femoral artery, and 1:1 diastolic augmentation was begun. His heart rate at this time was 118 and augmentation was inadequate. So counterpulsation was raised to a 1:2 ratio. This worked much better. Mr. Levinthal's condition improved slightly, and his urine output rose to 25 ml/hour. His heart rate came down to 100, so the balloon ratio was set back to a 1:1 ratio with better response. PO_2 remained around 85 mm Hg, and pH improved to 7.37. At this time, mean PA was 26 mm Hg.

Mr. Levinthal was receiving digoxin 0.25 mg daily and heparin 2000 units I.V. q2h. On the 4th day on IABP, he needed lidocaine infusion for multifocal PVCs but these subsided without recurrence. Dopamine was gradually withdrawn and discontinued on the 5th day of IABP. His vital signs remained fairly stable.

By the 7th day on IABP, Mr. Levinthal was weaned from the ventilator to oxygen by face mask at FIO_2, 50%. His BP was 110/60 with augmented diastolic pressure of 110 mm Hg. Heart rate was stable at 95 to 100; respiration, 26. He was slightly confused and disoriented. Blood gas determinations remained good. But Mr. Levinthal was still balloon-dependent. Weaning began on the 9th day of IABP with 1:2 augmentation ratio. He continued to improve and was transferred out of CCU a week later.

Some advances have been made in treating cardiogenic shock, but the main goal is still prevention by early detection of pump failure. Recent investigations have examined the theory that pump failure actually results from the infarction itself and the inflammatory and chemical changes that flow from it. For example, we know that the amines released in response to the occlusion cause most of the damage that follows (tissue destruction and clot formation). Experiments are now being done with such drugs as hyaluronidase and anti-inflammatories to see if they can prevent extension of infarction. Streptokinase, at one time an experimental treatment, has been proven to decrease the infarction size.

Ventricular aneurysm: Risk of embolism

When massive infarction destroys a large section of the left ventricle, the necrotic muscle can be reduced to a thin layer of fibrous tissue. When this thin layer dilates under the high pressure from the ventricular wall, it forms a separate noncontractile sac. Such an aneurysm is common in the anterior portion of the left ventricle (the area supplied by the anterior descending coronary artery) but may also occur posteriorly. Depending on size, you can see such an aneurysm on an X-ray as a definite bulge in the left ventricle. On palpation, you may feel a definite bulge in the precordium during systole.

In patients with ventricular aneurysm, stasis within the aneurysm can cause mural thrombi and systemic embolization. So check peripheral pulses regularly as well as the color and temperature of the extremities. Report hypotension immediately. Also watch for changes in the sensorium that may herald a CVA.

What confirms a suspected ventricular aneurysm? Several tests can confirm it: echocardiography, radioisotopic myocardial imaging, and ventriculography at cardiac catheterization.

Most patients who undergo resection of a ventricular aneurysm simultaneously have coronary bypass graft (see

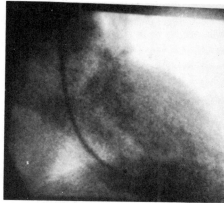

Aneurysm in the ventricle
A severe heart attack that destroys a large section of the left ventricle can produce a ventricular aneurysm like the one here. Necrotic tissue reduces to a thin sheath of fibrous tissue. High pressure in the ventricular wall causes this tissue to dilate. It then becomes a noncontractile sac, separate from the ventricle.

Most aneurysms are located in the anterior portion of the left ventricle, an area supplied by the anterior descending coronary artery. But they can be found in the posterior portion as well.

Depending on the size, you may be able to see an aneurysm on a chest X-ray. If it's visible, you'll see a suspicious bulge in the area of the left ventricle. A patient with a ventricular aneurysm may have persistent tachycardia, arrhythmias, intractable heart failure, and anginal pain that doesn't abate with nitrates.

Chapter 7). Without such resection, their prognosis depends on prevention of subsequent infarctions and congestive heart failure. Ventricular aneurysm can sometimes enlarge, but this is extremely rare.

Cardiac tamponade: Extreme emergency

Any fluid or blood in the pericardium limits ventricular ability to fill during diastole. If 150 to 200 ml of blood accumulates quickly in this closed membranous sac, it's a medical emergency — cardiac tamponade. The ventricle is so compressed that it can't eject forcefully, cardiac output falls, and the patient dies as the ventricle becomes too small to fill.

You'll see tamponade most often after open-heart surgery. Rarely, you'll see it after ventricular rupture, a complication of MI: When it occurs, it usually does so in the first week after infarction. Its cause is not well understood. There are usually no warning signs. A large perforation is, of course, immediately fatal. Sometimes, a smaller one leaves enough circulation to sustain a patient until he can get to the operating room for surgical repair. The clinical signs of cardiac tamponade may include falling blood pressure and shock syndrome, a rise in CVP, increased jugular vein distention, cyanosis, pulsus paradoxus, and faint heart sounds.

A conscious patient may describe such a slow perforation as a sharp or tearing pain over the precordium (not substernal, like angina). He reports that such pain varies with posture or respiration. In patients with such slow perforations, X-rays may show an enlarging cardiac shadow before clinical signs develop, but this is rare. Almost always, the onset of tamponade is sudden and catastrophic.

Cardiac tamponade needs immediate relief via pericardiocentesis or sternotomy. If the patient can't be moved to an O.R., sternotomy may be performed at the bedside using a thoracotomy tray. Have sterile equipment and blood available for rapid transfusion. Assemble emergency resuscitation equipment, including sterile internal defibrillator paddles at the bedside. Monitor the patient's EKG, CVP, and arterial pressure. There's usually no time for chest X-rays before sternotomy unless the tamponade has had a slow onset. However, as a temporary medical treatment (before pericardiocentesis or sternotomy can be done), simple intravenous infusion of fluid can be lifesaving. A rapid I.V. infusion

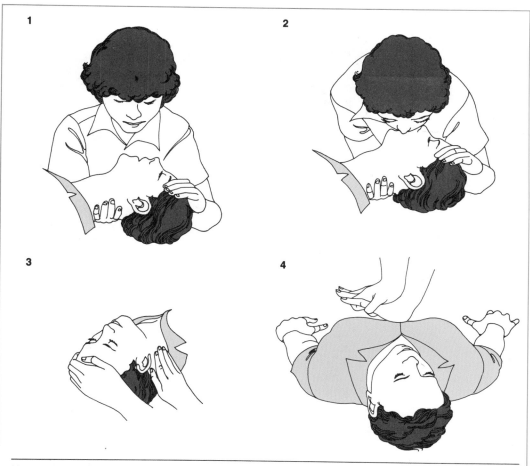

1

2

3

4

Success with CPR

External cardiac massage and artificial ventilation must begin within 4 to 6 minutes after cardiac arrest or irreversible brain damage will develop. To perform cardiopulmonary resuscitation (CPR) properly, you must receive instruction from a qualified instructor. These pictures merely illustrate the four basic steps of life support:

1. If the patient is unconscious, tilt his head back to relieve tongue obstruction and open his airway.

2. If he doesn't breathe spontaneously, begin artificial ventilation using a mouth-to-mouth or mouth-to-nose technique. Deliver several full breaths in quick succession.

3. Check his carotid artery for a pulse. If his neck is injured, feel instead for a femoral pulse.

4. If you can't feel a pulse, begin CPR immediately. Establish the correct position, and begin downward compressions, depressing the sternum 1½ to 2 inches. Maintain a rhythm of 80

compressions per minute if you are alone and 60 per minute if you are working with someone else.

Consider resuscitation efforts effective if you observe the following signs:

• constriction of the pupils
• carotid and femoral pulsations with each cardiac compression
• blinking upon stimulation of the eyelid
• breathing that begins spontaneously
• movement and struggling
• decreased cyanosis.

may allow the ventricle to fill enough to maintain reasonable cardiac output until the surgeon comes. So, if you suspect cardiac tamponade, start an I.V. infusion of 5% dextrose in water immediately.

During sternotomy, the mediastinum is cleared of blood and clots, allowing the ventricle full space for expansion and contraction. The patient's improvement is dramatic: immediate decrease in CVP, rise in blood pressure, and disappearance of cyanosis. After the sternum is closed, the patient should have prophylactic antibiotics.

Postoperatively, such patients need meticulous care of chest tubes. For the first several hours, milk and drain the chest tubes every 15 minutes to prevent clots from blocking drainage. Record the amount drained, noting whether it is sanguineous or serosanguineous. Report any sudden tachycardia, unexplained hypotension, or sudden cessation of chest drainage. Keep a Fogarty catheter handy to unclog a chest drain.

Pericardiocentesis is no less dangerous. Its risks include sudden death by laceration of a coronary artery or ventricular fibrillation, so keep emergency drugs and resuscitation equipment available. A large-bore needle is introduced into the pericardium through the skin to the left of the xiphoid process. An EKG lead attached to this needle identifies contact with the heart surface, decreasing the chance of injury to the myocardium. Repeated aspirations may be necessary and the patient may still need surgery to complete the evacuation.

After pericardiocentesis, watch for arrhythmias, such as PVCs, which may follow needle trauma.

Remember these important points when caring for a patient who's at risk of cardiac complications:

1. Watch for symptoms of cardiogenic shock: cold, clammy skin; pallor; cyanosis; mental confusion or lethargy; urine ouput less than 20 ml/hour; and a systolic blood pressure below 80 mm Hg.

2. During Swan-Ganz catheter insertion, monitor the EKG for ventricular irritability.

3. Be aware that a properly titrated dopamine drip (1 ampul of dopamine mixed in 250 or 500 ml dextrose 5% in water) increases mesenteric cerebral and renal blood flow and improves cardiac output by increasing preload and decreasing afterload.

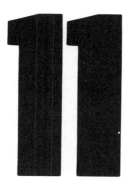

Inflammatory Heart Diseases
Four most common

BY MARY M. CANOBBIO, RN, BSN

INFLAMMATORY DISEASES of the heart were once nearly always lethal. Antibiotics have made them much less so and, in fact, much less prevalent. But they do still occur. They still produce life-threatening changes in the heart muscle and its structures — changes that are often difficult to recognize and to treat. To improve your own ability to deal with inflammatory diseases of the heart, you may want to review the most common ones: myocarditis, bacterial endocarditis, pericarditis, and rheumatic heart disease.

Myocarditis
Myocarditis denotes an infiltration of the myocardial cells by bacteria or viruses. These pathogens can cause myocardial damage by inciting toxic reactions or inflammatory response.

Myocarditis can occur after infection with almost any pathogen. For example, infection with group B-Coxsackie virus can induce myocarditis in neonates and infants. Some pathogens that can induce myocarditis include: bacteria *(Clostridium diphtheriae, S. pneumoniae);* viruses *(Coxsackie group B);* protozoas *(Trypanosoma cruzi,* the major cause of Chagas' diseases in South America); and fungi *(His-*

Pathology of myocarditis
In myocarditis, myocardial fibers disintegrate and diffuse throughout the myocardium, along with infiltrated lymphocytes. Certain pathogens, usually bacteria, may form localized microabscesses in the interstitium; viruses directly cause inflammation and necrosis of the myocardium. Toxins, such as the endotoxin of typhoid fever, may also produce inflammation as an allergic response. These changes may be localized or widespread.

toplasma capsulatum or *candida*). But infections are not the only cause of myocarditis. Secondary causes of myocarditis include rheumatic fever and other diseases that produce myocardial inflammation (such as bacterial endocarditis), toxic chemicals, or excessive radiation exposure.

What symptoms?

During the acute phase, the symptoms are systemic: fever, malaise, arthralgias, and fatigue. The patient may also have precordial discomfort typical of pericarditis or of angina. Other symptoms vary according to the extent of myocardial infiltration and may include tachycardia (unrelated to fever), hypotension, and symptoms of congestive failure. On auscultation, you may find a soft first heart sound, gallop rhythm, or systolic murmur (suggesting ventricular dilatation and mitral regurgitation). EKGs may show conduction disturbance (particularly prolonged P-R interval and ST-T wave changes), but these are often nonspecific for myocarditis.

Treatment of myocarditis includes bed rest during the acute stages and management of symptoms with diuretics, digitalis, and salt restriction for heart failure, and antiarrhythmics, as needed (which call for careful monitoring). Patients with viral myocarditis are very sensitive to digitalis and should have the short-acting forms, such as digoxin (Lanoxin). Generally, your nursing care is the same as that for any patient with an acute infection or congestive heart failure. Check for signs of cardiovascular deterioration. Assess breath sounds, vital signs, and central venous pressures frequently. Watch urine output. Report an output less than 30 ml/hr to the doctor. Also report any weight gain (worsening edema).

Bacterial endocarditis

Endocarditis means an acute or subacute bacterial (or fungal) invasion of the endocardium, heart valves, or valve prosthesis. Endocarditis is usually classified by the causative organism and clinical findings. Acute endocarditis is usually attributed to *Staphylococcus aureus* or pneumococcus; subacute bacterial endocarditis (SBE), to *Streptococcus viridans*.

Endocardial pathogens may enter via the skin or respiratory, gastrointestinal, or genitourinary tracts. These pathogens take hold most easily in patients with lowered endocardial resistance (patients with infections after congenital or rheumatic heart disease, or those recovering from open heart surgery, especially if they have prosthetic valve replacement and a history of drug abuse). It's crucial to use aseptic technique when changing surgical dressings. Patients with normal valves who have been infected via dental sepsis (*Streptococcus viridans* is common in the mouth) tend to be unusually vulnerable to bacterial infection in general. Who gets bacterial endocarditis? About half of all patients with bacterial endocarditis have a history of rheumatic fever.

Endocardial pathogens typically settle on the cardiac valves (often the mitral or aortic). Characteristically, they first infiltrate the contact aspect of the cusps but eventually extend through their full thickness. These bacterial colonies multiply by platelet and fibrin aggregation and set up an inflammatory vegetative process. Eventually these bulky vegetations prevent proper alignment of the valve cusps, producing poor closure and incompetence. The result may be scarring, retraction of leaflets, and ensuing insufficiency. These vegetations also have a tendency to dislodge and embolize.

Symptoms sometimes specific

The patient with endocarditis has a history of chronic fever — usually low-grade and intermittent. Depending on the virulence of the organism involved, the patient may also experience nocturnal sweats and chills, malaise, easy fatigue, anorexia, or arthralgia. These nonspecific symptoms often lead to studies for "fever of unknown origin," unless certain diagnostic findings (petechiae, Osler's nodes, splinter hemorrhages over nail beds, murmurs [a sign of aortic or mitral disease], and splenomegaly) point clearly to bacterial endocarditis. In elderly patients, a CVA with fever due to cerebral embolus from an infected valve may be the *first* sign of endocarditis.

What laboratory findings to expect? Blood cultures are positive for pathogens in 80% to 90% of patients. Other laboratory findings include an elevated sedimentation rate (90%) with slight leukocytosis and anemia (in SBE). Echocardiograms help to evaluate the extent of valvular damage. Electrocardiograms are generally not diagnostically helpful, but certain arrhythmias (such as atrial fibrillation) do point to valvular disease. Since none of these tests is specific for bacterial endocarditis, an accurate medical (and dental) history is

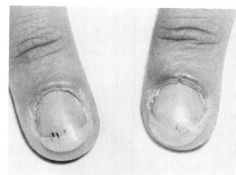

Signs of bacterial endocarditis
Endocarditis often produces a persistent low-grade fever, fatigue, and anorexia, which may be mistaken for symptoms of flu. Certain physical findings of bacterial endocarditis, however, can help pinpoint the correct diagnosis:
 • Petechiae usually found in the oral mucosa, conjunctiva, upper chest, and lower extremities
 • Tender, raised erythematous lesions found on the fingers and toe pads, known as Osler's nodes
 • Nontender splinter hemorrhages over the nail beds, as seen above
 • Murmurs, a sign of mitral or aortic disease, which occur in 85% of these cases
 • Pain in the left upper quadrant due to splenomegaly

Dangerous growth
This drawing shows the growth of
vegetations that is characteristic
of endocarditis. These
vegetations, composed of fibrin,
red cells, and platelets, settle
most commonly on the aortic and
mitral valves and can dislodge,
causing life-threatening emboli.

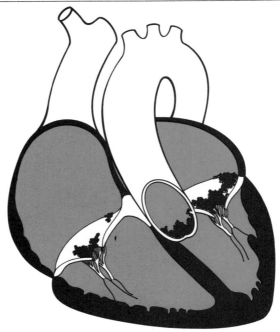

crucial for diagnosis.

Major complications of endocarditis include emboli from dislodged vegetations (which cause vascular accidents); nephritis, renal infarcts, and uremia; and heart failure (from severe valvular damage). Vital signs are the earliest clue to complications, so watch for changes in the temperature and respirations, and monitor the apical pulse to detect changes in heart rhythm and rate.

Managing endocarditis
Patients hospitalized with endocarditis are often very sick at admission. Typically, they are dehydrated and anorexic and show severe weight loss. They may need parenteral fluids. Because they have fever, remember to encourage oral fluid intake, too. Also keep track of their nutritional state; offer frequent small meals — likely to be more acceptable than large ones. Finally, remember that these patients need emotional support since their illness requires long-term hospitalization. As they begin to feel less acutely ill, they tend to become bored, depressed, angry, and frustrated; they need special support at such times.

Treatment aims to eradicate the infection; prevent cardiac damage and complications; treat the cardiac problems due to the inflammation; replace damaged valves when indicated; and finally, prevent spread or recurrence of infection.

Eradicating the infection obviously requires identification of the infecting pathogen, followed by appropriate antibiotic treatment. Endocarditis after penicillinase-producing staphylococcal infection calls for a penicillinase-resistant antibiotic given intravenously over a 6 to 8 week period. Such drugs include: methicillin (Staphcillin) 16-20 g/day; oxacillin (Prostaphlin) 4-6 g/day; or cephalothin (Keflin) 10-14 g/day. If the pathogen is *Streptococcus viridans*, or a non-penicillinase-producing staphylococcus, the best drug is intravenous penicillin-G potassium (usual dose in adults, 10 to 12 million units daily for 4 to 6 weeks). Remember to watch the serum potassium level in patients who need large doses of penicillin-G potassium. Such patients need routine assessment of renal function (BUN and creatinine). For patients allergic to penicillin, cephalothin (Keflin) and vancomycin (Vancocin) are effective substitutes. Some patients allergic to penicillin are also allergic to the cephalosporins.

In 10 to 20% of patients with endocarditis, blood cultures come up negative even in repeated tests. Such patients may receive aqueous penicillin-G, 12-20 million units daily I.V., for 4 weeks, with streptomycin, 1 g daily, during the first 10 days of treatment.

Preventing cardiac damage and complications depends almost entirely on early diagnosis and treatment. Unfortunately, many patients go untreated for a long time, until progressive weakness, persistent fever, and general malaise force them to seek help. When finally hospitalized, they are usually quite debilitated, and dehydrated, and have some signs of cardiac complications. Watch for early signs of cardiac involvement: irregular pulse, tachycardia, chest discomfort, dyspnea on exertion, and any signs of heart failure and emboli. To help such patients recover, monitor their activity and promote plenty of rest; see that bedridden patients are turned frequently; teach coughing and deep-breathing exercises, and provide antiembolic stockings. Auscultate breath sounds carefully to detect early signs of failure or secondary respiratory infections.

Preventing recurring infection requires prophylactic use of

Valve replacement
Here you can see a prosthetic
Starr Edwards mitral valve in
place.

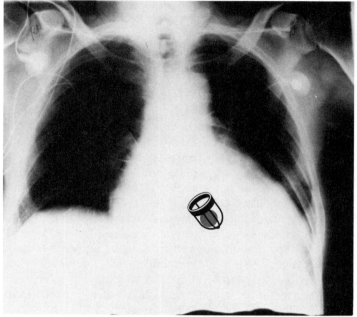

antibiotics during procedures known to cause bacteremia in high-risk patients. Such patients include those with congenital heart lesions, rheumatic fever, known valvular disease, or cardiac murmurs. They need prophylactic antibiotics and special care during any procedures likely to cause transient bacteremia (dental work and any genitourinary or gastrointestinal procedures). They should seek medical treatment for persistent sore throats or any bacterial infection like boils on the skin.

When cardiac problems persist
What if, despite antibiotic therapy, the patient continues to show signs of cardiac failure, valvular damage, deteriorating cardiac function or persistent bacteremia? Then he may need evaluation for surgical correction (such as prosthetic replacement of the mitral or aortic valves). Whenever possible, surgery is deferred until after the sepsis is controlled. The decision for surgery is often difficult because these patients are typically poor surgical risks — especially when they are elderly, or have heart failure, or severely incompetent valves. Consider Mr. Jarvis.

Mr. Jacob Jarvis, a 31-year-old jeweler, was hospitalized for treatment of subacute bacterial endocarditis. He had been treating himself at home for what he thought was the flu. At admission, he had fever, dyspnea, and general malaise. Physical exam revealed a Grade III/VI systolic murmur at the apex, with engorged neck veins and bilateral rales over the lung fields. He had scattered petechiae on his upper chest; he did not have Osler's nodes or splinter hemorrhages.

Blood culture was positive for streptococcus, so he received penicillin (10 million units daily, I.V.) for 4 weeks. However, he continued to deteriorate, showing daily, progressive weakness, weight loss, dyspnea on exertion, and increasing signs of heart failure. After an echocardiogram and cardiac catheterization disclosed vegetations on the mitral valve, he was evaluated for possible valve replacement. The surgeon postponed this until heart failure and sepsis were relieved.

After 4 more weeks of treatment, Mr. Jarvis improved enough for mitral valve replacement. He had a successful porcine valve replacement and an uneventful postoperative recovery. He was discharged in good condition within 10 days of surgery.

Pericarditis

Pericarditis refers to inflammation of the pericardium. It occurs in acute and chronic forms. Acute pericarditis can be fibrinous or effusive, with purulent, serous, or hemorrhagic exudate; chronic constrictive pericarditis is characterized by dense fibrous pericardial thickening, with or without calcification that impairs cardiac function. Common causes of pericarditis include: infections (bacterial, viral, or fungal); systemic disease (rheumatoid arthritis, systemic lupus erythematosus, and myocardial infarction); trauma to the chest or myocardium; neoplasm (lymphomas); high-dose radiation to the chest; uremia; and drugs, such as hydralazine or procainamide.

In pericarditis, the inflammation commonly involves the lower portion of the parietal pericardium, an area that carries pain receptors. So patients with pericarditis commonly complain of chest pain, especially...
- when they move the torso
- when they cough or take a deep breath
- when they are recumbent.

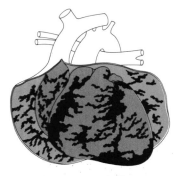

The rigid heart
One kind of pericarditis, called chronic constrictive pericarditis, causes a gradual increase in systemic venous pressure and produces symptoms similar to those of chronic right-sided heart failure.

Such pain may be dull or sharp; precordial or substernal; and can radiate to the neck, trapezius, shoulder, and down the arms. Since this pain pattern is similar to that of myocardial infarction, careful assessment is crucial.

The most helpful clue? Pericardial pain usually changes with respiration and a change in body position. It diminishes when the patient sits up and leans forward (sitting up pulls the heart away from the diaphragmatic pleura of the lung).

Another classic sign is the pericardial friction rub. You can hear this sound by listening with your stethoscope over the patient's apical area. This sound is due to myocardial movement during atrial and ventricular systole and ventricular diastole, which rubs the pericardium against the diaphragmatic pleura. Listen for an intermittent, transient, "to and fro" sound much like sandpaper rubbing together.

Depending on the underlying cause, the patient may have associated symptoms: fever, dyspnea, chills, fatigue, or tachycardia. Therapy of pericarditis aims to remove the underlying cause and relieve symptoms. It usually includes reassurance and support, bed rest, aspirin for fever and pain, and sometimes, steroids.

Patients may also develop pericardial effusion. If fluid accumulates rapidly between the pericardium and myocardium, cardiac compression and tamponade could occur. Watch for decreased blood pressure, tachycardia, cool clammy skin, distended neck veins, elevated CVP, and pulsus paradoxus. If you see any of these symptoms, notify the doctor *immediately*. The patient will need a pericardial tap, a pleuropericardial window, or pericardiectomy to save his life. Serum lab studies may show an elevated leukocyte count and erythrocyte sedimentation rate (ESR). On EKG you may see low voltage of the P-QRS-T complex with S-T segment elevation and T wave inversion. However, these changes are nonspecific. More helpful are an echocardiogram to determine the amount of accumulating fluid and X-rays to show an enlarged heart or pericardial effusion.

Rheumatic heart disease
Rheumatic heart disease denotes the cardiac involvement that follows rheumatic fever. Rheumatic fever, generally considered a childhood disease, has become much less common during the last 30 years because of the successful use of an-

tibiotics against streptococcal infections. But it does still occur. Rheumatic fever usually develops 2 to 3 weeks after acute pharyngitis due to hemolytic streptococci. It's an inflammatory disease caused by abnormal tissue reaction to an autoimmune mechanism. It affects various organs and tissues, and typically produces polyarthritis (usually of larger joints), subcutaneous nodules, and carditis (an acute inflammatory reaction of the heart muscle or pericardium). Roughly a third of the children with rheumatic fever have some signs of carditis during the acute stage. Such carditis can cause irreversible heart damage. Fortunately, in most children, it heals completely or leaves only insignificant scarring.

Clinical signs delayed

Remember, there's usually a long latent period between the first attack of rheumatic fever and a full-blown case of rheumatic heart disease. The patient usually lives a normal life without a hint of a problem. He may be told he has a murmur, but it causes him no difficulty. At age 30 or 40, cardiac symptoms may begin.

Mrs. Grant, a 32-year-old mother of two young children had rheumatic fever when she was 12. She had no symptoms after that until she was 31. Then she began to feel shortness of breath and slight chest discomfort after exercising, which she attributed to her age and lack of regular exercise. But when her symptoms recurred even with minimal exercise, she became worried and sought medical help. A thorough medical history and physical findings typical of valvular disease led to a diagnosis of rheumatic heart disease (see insert).

Rheumatic heart disease can mean extensive pathologic changes. During the acute inflammatory stages, rheumatic heart disease can affect all layers of the heart muscle producing: myocarditis (cardiac failure and hypertrophy may result); pericarditis (causing the surface of the heart to become reddened and rough, often with a fibrinous exudate); and endocarditis (involving the endocardium and valves, usually of the left side of the heart). The valve leaflets become edematous and inflamed, and vegetations appear along the closure line. The principal valvular sequelae of rheumatic heart disease are mitral and/or aortic regurgitation and mitral stenosis. Regurgitation results when inflammation and edema of the leaflets produce retraction of the leaflets and cusps; stenosis results

Signs and symptoms of valve disorders

MITRAL REGURGITATION
• Systolic murmur heard best at the apex and transmitted to the axilla, left sternal border, and base of the heart
• EKG — P wave abnormalities, atrial fibrillation, PACs
• Increasing fatigue and dyspnea.

MITRAL STENOSIS
• Diastolic murmur heard best over the apex, and transmitted to the axilla, epigastrium, left sternal border
• EKG — notched and peaked P waves, atrial fibrillation
• Increased fatigue with decreased exercise tolerance and dyspnea.

AORTIC REGURGITATION
• Decrescendo diastolic murmur of blowing quality heard best over left lower sternal border
• Loudest in aortic area and transmitted to the axilla and left sternal border
• EKG — left ventricular hypertrophy
• Dyspnea on exertion, bounding pulse with a rapid rise and fall; deMusset's sign, widened arterial pulse pressure.

when the leaflets become rigid with calcified cusp adhesions.

No laboratory test points specifically to rheumatic heart disease. However, some useful tests identify infective pathogens and measure inflammation via leukocyte count, sedimentation rate, and C-reactive protein. Echocardiograms identify the presence and severity of any valvular damage. Cardiac catheterization evaluates valvular disease and overall cardiac function in terms of left ventricular function and cardiac output.

Many patients with rheumatic heart disease never develop serious problems and lead normal lives. However, a certain percentage develop recurrent infections or signs of heart failure. So medical management depends on the severity of valvular disease, the patient's symptoms, and any complications (SBE or heart failure). Treatment aims to relieve cardiac symptoms and sepsis (via antibiotics, low-sodium diet, diuretics, digitalis, beta-adrenergic blockers, and antiarrhythmic agents).

The same criteria determine surgical intervention. Is the patient symptomatic or septic? If so, how severely? Severe cases may require surgery, despite the risk, because of the danger of spontaneous rupture of the papillary muscles and the threat of embolism or intractable congenital heart failure.

After valve surgery, patients need detailed information on diet, exercise, medications, and special precautions against infections. Make sure they understand their need for prophylactic antibiotic treatment during any dental work or gastrointestinal or genitourinary procedures. Stress that they must remember to tell all dentists and doctors who treat them about their valve replacement.

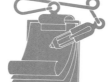

Remember these important points when dealing with inflammatory heart diseases:
1. Stay alert for symptoms of acute myocarditis: fever, malaise, arthralgias, and fatigue.
2. Advise a patient with rheumatic heart disease to be sure she receives prophylactic antibiotics before dental, genitourinary, and obstetric procedures to minimize the risk of endocarditis.
3. Be aware that echocardiograms identify vegetations in about half of all endocarditis cases.
4. Suspect endocarditis in a patient with blood cultures positive for pathogens and an elevated sedimentation rate with slight leukocytosis and anemia.

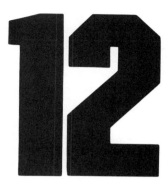

12

Cardiomyopathy
Mysterious dysfunction

BY KATHLEEN A. DRACUP, RN, MN

TOM, A TALL, HANDSOME FRESHMAN from the local university really stood out among the much older patients in the Coronary Observation Unit. In his street clothes and tennis shoes, he looked and moved like the athlete he was. The only clue to his patient status was the Holter recording device strapped over his shoulder. What was an apparently healthy person doing in the COU? Three mornings ago, he had been jogging in the park. The next thing he remembered, he was lying on the ground looking into the faces of two paramedics and several fellow joggers. While running, he had suddenly collapsed. Luckily, the woman jogging behind him happened to be an anesthesiologist, who immediately started cardiopulmonary resuscitation. The paramedics, who arrived quickly, found him in ventricular fibrillation, which they successfully converted. He was awake and asking questions as they placed him on a stretcher and into the ambulance. Now, after 3 days of diagnostic tests, the doctors were telling him he had heart disease.

At the same time, Captain Morgan lay dying in the Coronary Care Unit nearby. A retired Air Force pilot, he had a long history of alcohol abuse. After multiple admissions during the past year for congestive heart failure, he was now unresponsive to treatment.

A third patient, Fernanda Moreno, a 38-year-old mother of a 6-week-old infant, was hospitalized in the CCU because she was having trouble breathing. She couldn't understand why she should still feel so weak when her recent labor and delivery had gone so well.

These three patients — seemingly so different — shared the same diagnosis: cardiomyopathy. The disparity in their ages and conditions truly reflects the nature of this disease. Actually, it's not one disease, but a group of diseases involving pathology of the heart muscle. It can affect young and old alike. Its cause is usually unknown and its prognosis, poor. Therefore, treatment is usually palliative, not curative. Patients with cardiomyopathy have to deal with a shortened life span, and with numerous changes in life-style (diet, medication, and exercise) demanded by medical treatment.

What is it?

Cardiomyopathy simply means heart (cardio) muscle (myo) disease (pathy). Other terms have also been used: myocardiopathy, idiopathic myocardial hypertrophy, idiopathic cardiomegaly, and primary myocardial disease, to name but a few. All of these terms describe a group of diseases which affect the myocardium without affecting other cardiovascular structures like the heart valves or the coronary arteries. Many cases of heart failure are now known to result from cardiomyopathy, rather than coronary artery obstruction or rheumatic myocarditis, or rheumatic valvular disease.

Much is still unknown about cardiomyopathy. But three of its features are almost universally accepted:

• The cause of the disease is unknown or unusual.

• It involves a disorder of the heart muscle, sometimes associated with endocardial and/or pericardial involvement.

• Cardiomegaly and heart failure predominate.

Cardiomyopathy may be primary (when the heart alone is involved) or secondary (when other organs are involved as well). Some examples of secondary cardiomyopathy: hemochromatosis (a metabolic disease characterized by excessive deposition of iron in the myocardium and other tissues); sarcoidosis; amyloidosis (which affects connective tissues); and certain neurological disorders (muscular dystrophy).

THREE KINDS OF CARDIOMYOPATHY

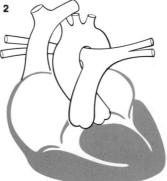 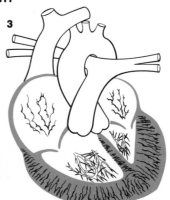

1. CONGESTIVE — Congestive cardiomyopathy is the most common form. It involves extensive damage to the myofibrils, interference with myocardial metabolism, and gross dilation of the heart. In other forms of heart disease that produce such dilation (such as aortic regurgitation), hypertrophy of the ventricular muscle keeps pace with the dilation. This combination of hypertrophy and dilation creates an enlarged heart, but effective ventricular function persists until the late stage of the disease. However, in congestive cardiomyopathy, there's little or no hypertrophy. The heart takes on a globular shape and contracts poorly during its ejection phase (systole). In congestive cardiomyopathy, the heart ejects only 20% of the blood in the left ventricle (compared to 70% in the normal heart). Because of this inability to pump effectively, a large volume of blood remains in the left ventricle after systole. Consequently, congestive heart failure soon follows: first, left-sided (shortness of breath, orthopnea, and dyspnea on exertion), then right-sided (dependent edema, liver

engorgement, and anasarca). Patients with congestive cardiomyopathy are usually hospitalized with heart failure, arrhythmias, and embolic phenomena. Typically, they have a large heart, gallop rhythms, and valvular insufficiency.

Many of the congestive cardiomyopathies are probably not primary myocardial disorders at all, but result from destruction of myocardial cells by toxic, infectious, or metabolic agents. Such agents include alcohol, certain viruses, endocrine and electrolyte disorders, and nutritional deficiencies.

2. HYPERTROPHIC — This cardiomyopathy may be inherited. It's a bizarre muscular hypertrophy that affects all the heart muscles but is most prominent in the ventricular septum. Unlike the congestive form, it doesn't produce dilation. The overgrowth of heart muscle makes the ventricular walls rigid, increasing the resistance to blood entering from the left atrium. With this condition, cardiac output can be normal, high, or low. If cardiac output is high or normal, the patient may have no symptoms

and may remain undiagnosed for years. Eventually, though, cardiac function deteriorates.

Patients with hypertrophic cardiomyopathy have inadequate ventricular filling and may have decreased mitral valve compliance. This combination results from the hypertrophy of the left ventricular septum and papillary muscles of the mitral valve. Muscle hypertrophy may affect the outflow tract, which affects the systolic function of the heart.

3. RESTRICTIVE — This rarest form may be easily misdiagnosed as constrictive pericarditis. Restrictive cardiomyopathy involves an infiltration of the myocardium, endocardium, and subendocardium with fibroelastic tissue, similar to that in amyloid disease. This infiltration makes the heart rigid, so it doesn't distend well in diastole or contract completely in systole. The end result is low cardiac output and, eventually, the symptoms of congestive failure (dyspnea, orthopnea, edema, liver engorgement, and anasarca).

A fourth category, obliterative, is extremely rare among people in temperate climates.

Three forms of cardiomyopathy

Based on their physiological and clinical signs, heart muscle diseases can be divided into three major groups: congestive, hypertrophic, and restrictive (see page 127). A fourth category, obliterative, is extremely rare in temperate climates like the United States, and we will not discuss it here.

Many of the congestive cardiomyopathies are secondary disorders, the result of myocardial destruction by toxic, infectious, or metabolic agents. Occasionally, they may result from ischemic heart disease. Usually, however, patients with congestive cardiomyopathy have normal coronary arteries on arteriography.

One of the most commonly recognized toxic agents is *alcohol*, with or without malnutrition. Excessive ingestion of alcohol can produce severe congestive heart failure that tends to improve when the patient stops drinking, and recurs when he takes it up again. But not everyone who abuses alcohol develops alcoholic cardiomyopathy. Probably individual differences and susceptibilities, combined with other risk factors, explain this discrepancy.

Viruses may also produce congestive cardiomyopathy. Many investigators are studying a possible link between the viral infection of myocarditis and later development of congestive cardiomyopathy. The viruses currently implicated are coxsackievirus B, poliovirus, and influenza.

Metabolic cardiomyopathies follow *endocrine* and *electrolyte* disorders and nutritional deficiences. For example, hyperthyroidism, pheochromocytoma, beriberi (thiamine deficiency) and kwashiorkor (protein deficiency) have been associated with congestive cardiomyopathy.

One form of congestive cardiomyopathy does not fall neatly into any one of the above categories and is particularly poignant to deal with: postpartum or peripartum cardiomyopathy. It develops in some women in the last trimester or up to 5 months after delivery. Its cause is unknown, but is most common in multiparous women over 30. Treatment sometimes reverses this kind of cardiomegaly and congestive heart failure. If it does, these women can live on, and even have subsequent pregnancies without cardiac problems. But if cardiomegaly persists despite treatment, the prognosis is extremely poor.

In the United States, hypertrophic cardiomyopathy with

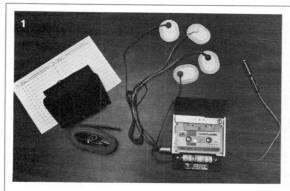

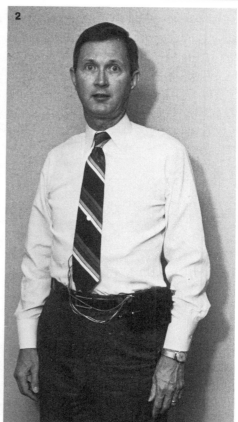

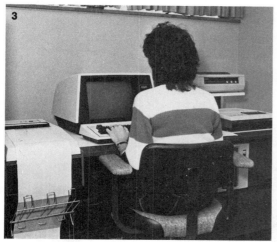

Key to the heart

Ambulatory electrocardiography, also known as Holter monitoring after Dr. Norman J. Holter who conceived and developed the process, enables a doctor to monitor as many as 100,000 cardiac cycles over a 24-hour period. The advantages of this method are many.

With very little equipment, the doctor can hook up a patient to one or more EKG leads. These record onto a portable cassette tape recorder (Figure 1) which the patient can wear easily.

The recorder should be connected to an EKG for test readings. After the hookup has been checked, the patient goes through a normal day (Figure 2) on the monitor. He is encouraged to try out those activities that bring on his symptoms, keeping a diary to record the exact times of symptoms, activities, and any drugs he takes so that their impact can be correlated with the EKG printouts. With the aid of a high-speed scanner (Figure 3), the doctor can review 24 hours of tape in 24 minutes, picking up important EKG changes.

Although not a substitute for CCU monitoring, the Holter monitor can catch a sporadic rhythm disturbance that an office or stress-test EKG might miss. It also saves the patient the time and expense of a hospital stay.

Holter monitoring has proved useful for patients recuperating from myocardial infarctions, those taking antiarrhythmic drugs, or those using pacemakers. It can catch rate, rhythm, and conduction abnormalities as well as cardiac responses to a normal environment. It is especially useful in diagnosing arrhythmias and the cause of CNS symptoms.

Ten common problems in cardiomyopathy patients

You can help a patient with cardiomyopathy by teaching him about his illness, what produces his symptoms, how to control them with medication, and how to pace his activities to avoid taxing his heart. His precarious condition may cause him severe psychiatric disturbances, so counsel him well and, when necessary, refer him for psychosocial intervention.

Expect to see:
1. dyspnea secondary to heart failure
2. syncope with ventricular outflow tract problems (in IHSS)
3. chest pain secondary to low cardiac output (in some patients only)
4. fatigue secondary to inadequate cardiac output and/or heart failure
5. anxiety (fear of sudden death)
6. depression or hopelessness
7. body image disturbance
8. role disturbance
9. forced dependency
10. poor cooperation with prescribed treatment

inadequate ventricular filling and decreased mitral valve compliance is called *radiopathic hypertrophic subaortic stenosis (IHSS)*.

Patients with IHSS may have angina pectoris, palpitations or arrhythmias, dyspnea, syncope, and, rarely, congestive heart failure. They have a medium-pitched systolic ejection murmur heard along the left sternal border and at the apex. Their peripheral pulse has a characteristic double impulse (pulsus bisferiens).

Many patients with IHSS remain asymptomatic for a long time. The very first sign of the disease may be cardiac arrest, although the reason for susceptibility to fatal arrhythmias is not clear. As the disease progresses, the atria become dilated and atrial fibrillation becomes common. In late stages, congestive heart failure occurs.

In restrictive cardiomyopathy, the heart becomes rigid so it doesn't adequately distend in diastole or contract in systole. Low cardiac output follows with its characteristic symptoms: easy fatigue, dyspnea on exertion, and symptoms of congestive heart failure. Fortunately, restrictive cardiomyopathy is extremely rare.

Diagnosis by testing

Diagnosis of cardiomyopathy is based on clinical findings and test results. Echocardiography can identify most cases of congestive and hypertrophic cardiomyopathies. For example, a positive echocardiogram shows increased thickness of the interventricular septum and abnormal motion of the anterior mitral leaflet during systole. Cardiac catheterization reveals elevated left ventricular end-diastolic pressure and, possibly, mitral insufficiency. The characteristic EKG changes include left ventricular hypertrophy, S-T segment and T wave abnormalities, left anterior hemiblock, ventricular arrhythmias, and possibly atrial fibrillation. Phonocardiography confirms an early systolic murmur.

Most treatment palliative

When cardiomyopathy stems from some known cause, such as alcohol or drugs, obviously the cause must be withdrawn. Of course, in alcoholic cardiomyopathy, removing the cause is not as easy as it sounds. But in most cases, the cause is unknown and, so, treatment is palliative rather than curative.

Overall, cardiomyopathy is a degenerative disease with a poor prognosis, but certain treatment does help, depending on the kind of cardiomyopathy.

In congestive cardiomyopathy, treatment aims to improve the heart's ability to function as a pump and to relieve symptoms of heart failure. Such treatment usually includes digitalis, diuretics, a low-sodium diet, and oxygen. If may also include steroids and prolonged bed rest.

In the last 5 years, vasodilators have been found effective in treating refractory heart failure in congestive cardiomyopathy. Their effectiveness has been attributed to the reduction of outflow (peripheral vascular) resistance. Possibly, vasodilators may also improve myocardial perfusion, which might be inadequate with dilated and hypertrophied muscle despite normal coronary arteries.

In the acutely ill patient, vasodilation can be achieved with intravenous infusion of sodium nitroprusside; later, it can be maintained with long-acting nitrates, hydralazine hydrochloride, prazosin hydrochloride, or captopril. These drugs relieve dyspnea and orthopnea by increasing cardiac output and decreasing pulmonary venous pressure. This treatment has given many former "cardiac cripples" new capabilities. After treatment with any of these drugs, some patients with severe and incapacitating heart disease become relatively symptom-free and able to resume activities long since abandoned. This treatment is still only palliative, but it does control congestive heart failure in such patients.

In hypertrophic cardiomyopathies, treatment aims to relax the ventricle and relieve obstruction of the outflow tract. Since many of these patients are diagnosed in their teens or twenties (Tom, the young athlete, had typical IHSS), exercise restriction, diet modification, and lifelong medication are crucial issues.

Surgical treatment has been tried with varying success. Ventricular myotomy (resection of the hypertrophied septum) and mitral valve replacement, alone or in conjunction with ventricular myotomy, have been tried. These techniques have noticeably eased outflow tract obstruction and have relieved symptoms, but surgical mortality is high (usually 10% to 20%). Because surgical intervention is only palliative and the prognosis so uncertain, such treatment is still considered experimental.

Medical treatment uses verapamil (Isoptin), a calcium blocker, and propranolol (Inderal), a beta-adrenergic blocker, which effectively reduce angina, syncope, dyspnea, and arrhythmias in patients with IHSS. When indicated, electrophysiology studies may be performed to determine the underlying cause and proper treatment of ventricular arrhythmias. Warn patients on drug therapy against stopping them abruptly. This can bring on a rebound of symptoms and sudden death.

In the end stage of the disease, atrial fibrillation usually develops. Digitalis and/or cardioversion can usually successfully convert the rhythm. Since there's a great risk of systemic embolism, the patient needs anticoagulants as long as he's in atrial fibrillation. In restrictive cardiomyopathies, treatment includes digitalis to improve contractility, diuretics and a low-sodium diet to reduce preload, and oral vasodilators (prazosin and hydralazine) to treat the intractable congestive failure. Monitor these patients carefully (especially blood pressure and urine output) when treatment with vasodilators begins. If acutely ill, they may need hemodynamic monitoring with the Swan-Ganz pulmonary catheter.

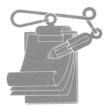

Remember these important points when caring for a patient with a cardiomyopathy:
1. Be able to differentiate between the three kinds of cardiomyopathies: congestive (extensive damage to the myofibrils, interference with myocardial metabolism, and gross heart dilation), hypertrophic (hypertrophy of the left ventricular septum and sometimes all the heart muscle), and restrictive (an infiltration of the myocardium, endocardium, and subendocardium with fibroelastic tissue).
2. Know that many cases of congestive cardiomyopathy are secondary disorders resulting from myocardial destruction by toxic (most commonly alcohol), infectious, or metabolic agents.
3. Suspect idiopathic hypertrophic subaortic stenosis in a patient with angina pectoris, palpitations or arrhythmias, dyspnea, syncope, and, possibly, congestive heart failure.
4. Consider echocardiography essential in diagnosing congestive and hypertrophic cardiomyopathy.
5. When caring for a congestive cardiomyopathy patient, give long-acting nitrates, hydralazine, prazosin, or captopril, as ordered, as well as diuretics, a low-sodium diet, and oxygen.

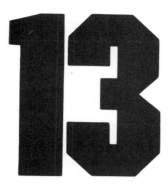

Pulmonary Embolism
Hazard of immobilization

BY M. SANDY WYPER, RN, MSN

PULMONARY EMBOLISM strikes young and old, men and women, in the hospital and on the street. In hospitalized patients, it is the most common pulmonary complication. To cope with this exceedingly common problem, you need to know what conditions make pulmonary embolism a likely complication...How to care for patients with an embolism.... Most important, you need to know what nursing measures can help prevent it.

Who gets it?

It's especially likely among immobilized patients; those recovering from surgery; patients with myocardial infarction, cerebrovascular accidents, congestive heart failure, fractures, and burns; and elderly patients with debilitating diseases. Mr. Andrews, a 69-year-old laborer, was recovering from a medullary stroke in the rehabilitation unit of a general hospital. Twenty days after admission, he awoke from an afternoon nap complaining of dyspnea and a dull, diffuse chest pain. His respirations were rapid but he was not cyanotic. His systolic blood pressure had fallen to 95 mm Hg. His nurse called a doctor, elevated the head of the bed 45 degrees, and started

What is pulmonary embolism?
It is any obstruction of the pulmonary vascular bed. Typically, a dislodged thrombus causes such obstruction, but it can be caused by any foreign substance.

Thromboembolism: Of the pulmonary emboli caused by a dislodged thrombi, 75% originate in the peripheral venous system (almost half of these in the deep veins of the lower extremities); 10% in pelvic veins; and 10% in the right heart chamber.

A *fat embolism* commonly follows fracture of long bones and other trauma such as closed-chest massage, burns, nephritis, infections, and liver disease (including that induced by alcoholism).

An *air embolism* may be caused by improper technique in administering intravenous infusions or any procedure in which air is injected into a body cavity.

Amniotic fluid emboli may follow complications of pregnancy including intrauterine fetal death and placenta previa. The amniotic fluid itself predisposes to deposition of fibrin throughout the venous system. Moreover, the solid contents of the fluid such as lipids and lanugo hair may embolize.

Tumor emboli, which may embolize from either primary or metastatic sites, probably occur more frequently than is generally thought.

oxygen by mask to relieve his dyspnea. She also started an I.V. to avoid difficulty later if his blood pressure continued to drop.

Physical examination showed that the chest was clear. But an EKG showed a rapid, regular heart rate of 150 beats/minute. The arrhythmia converted to normal sinus rhythm after administration of 3 mg of I.V. propranolol (Inderal) and the application of carotid sinus pressure. This response to treatment made paroxysmal atrial tachycardia the most likely diagnosis. The dyspnea and pain subsided within a few minutes. The only other notable finding was mild tenderness in the calf, which the patient said had been present for several months.

The attending staff considered several possible causes. A simple bout of arrhythmia that decreased cardiac output sufficiently to cause angina? A myocardial infarction? Both were possible, but pulmonary embolism was most likely in view of the calf pain and the patient's long immobilization.

Mr. Andrews was transferred to an actue medical unit for further evaluation. At the time of the transfer, his blood gases showed a low PO_2 (80) and a low PCO_2 (33). Mr. Andrews had a history of GI bleeding, so anticoagulant therapy was inadvisable without a certain diagnosis of pulmonary embolism. A lung scan showed a perfusion defect in the right lower lung field, which did not correlate with any abnormality on X-ray. This confirmed pulmonary embolism, and anticoagulant treatment was begun.

Mr. Andrews' pulmonary embolism was decidedly atypical in that it was immediately suspected and quickly confirmed. Generally, recognizing a pulmonary embolus is much more difficult. Fewer than half of pulmonary emboli are detected while the patient is alive! Consequently, prevention is doubly important. But to prevent most emboli, you must prevent the formation of thrombi.

What causes thrombi?
Three conditions predispose to thrombus formation: hypercoagulability of the blood; alterations in the integrity of blood vessel walls; and venous stasis (see page 160). Obviously, preventing thrombus formation requires prevention of these three conditions. Unfortunately, little can be done to prevent hypercoagulability.

To reduce the coagulability of the blood, anticoagulants are sometimes ordered. Because these drugs are not without risks, careful consideration's given before administering them.

You can do several things to minimize damage to vessel walls. First, of course, avoid venipuncture trauma by placing intravenous needles carefully. Also, avoid placing I.V.s in leg and pelvic veins, which have the greatest tendency to thrombus formation. Also minimize vessel wall damage associated with chronic conditions by frequently changing the patient's body position. Such changes shift pressure points and stimulate neural reflexes that help prevent venous distention and thus prevent pooling in dependent areas. Encourage patients who can move without help to do so often. Be sure they understand the dangers of remaining in one position too long or of allowing prolonged pressure on one area (as happens when sitting with legs crossed). Healthy people *automatically* change their body position at least every 30 minutes. So remember to help immobilized patients frequently. Never make patients wait for the minimum q2h turnings we often find on nursing care plans.

Venous stasis causes clots and also extends existing clots. Thus, it can complicate all other thrombus-associated conditions. Venous stasis is sometimes linked to obesity, congestive heart failure, and certain arrhythmias. But its most important predisposing factor is long-term immobility. In immobile patients like Mr. Andrews, bed rest decreases blood flow by approximately 50% because of the loss of muscle tone, which normally assists in pushing blood back to the heart. Immobilization also causes generalized vasodilation (from increased parasympathetic nervous system activity) and this, in turn, promotes pooling in dependent areas. Much can be done to prevent this major cause of thrombus formation. And you're usually the one who can do it. How to prevent thrombus formation?

Encourage ambulation

The trend toward early ambulation after surgery and to a limited extent after myocardial infarction has prevented venous stasis in many patients. To encourage early ambulation, you must explain the need for it to get the patient's cooperation. Encourage self-care, as prescribed, while keeping track of its effect on the patient's cardiovascular status and well-being. Continue to monitor the heart rate and watch for arrhythmia.

Hints on heparin

Heparin is commonly administered by I.V. intermittent bolus injection. Since it has a short half-life — about 60 minutes — never give bolus doses more often than every 4 hours. To check effectiveness, draw blood for the partial thromboplastin time (PTT) test half an hour before the next heparin dose is due. Adjust dosage to achieve a therapeutic level that is 2½ times the normal control, which is 35 to 45 seconds.

Continuous infusion produces less bleeding (an incidence 8 to 10 times lower) than bolus injections, but it needs close monitoring. Use an I.V. pump or controller to prevent inadvertent overdose by too fast an infusion. Or, use a 100-ml burette chamber and fill it hourly.

Don't delay giving heparin because blood isn't drawn in time or you haven't received lab results. Notify the doctor that heparin is due. If you can't reach him in 5 minutes, give the heparin on schedule and then try to reach the doctor and inform him why the blood wasn't drawn. Withhold heparin only if the patient has nosebleeds, ecchymoses, bloody urine, or other side effects. In that case, notify the doctor immediately.

Don't be alarmed if the doctor prescribes a high dose of heparin. Because pulmonary embolism decreases heparin's half-life, patients with this condition require a higher-than-normal initial dose.

Of course, policies vary from institution to institution, so make sure you know your own hospital's rules about heparin before using it.

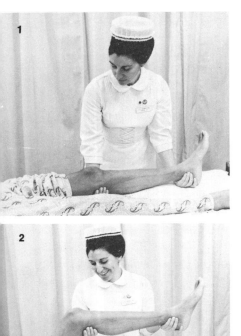

Bend and stretch
A bedridden patient needs
exercise to prevent venous stasis.
If he can't move, help him with
passive exercises.
   1. Place one hand under the
patient's knee and your other hand
on his heel.
   2. Lift his leg. Bend it at the
knee.

Don't allow the patient to exercise to the point of exhaustion.
(It's worth remembering that patients find using a bedside
commode much less exhausting than using a bedpan.)

Encourage exercise
Every nurse can glibly recite the maneuvers that supposedly
prevent venous stasis in the bedridden patient. But not nearly
so many practice these maneuvers with the required zeal.
Admittedly, teaching a reluctant patient to exercise properly
can be frustrating. And many nurses have been discouraged by
statements that the standard preventive measures do not really
decrease thrombus formation. If you have been discouraged
by such statements, you should know that a United States
Public Health Service report cites disability from immobilization as one of the top ten preventable health problems. This
report also suggests that these disabilities could probably be
reduced by 50 to 75%. That's strong support for vigorous
nursing measures.
   What nursing measures may be most effective? Because
over 75% of embolized thrombi originate in the main venous
channels of the lower leg, most preventive measures emphasize positioning and exercising of the legs, elastic stockings
or bandages, and deep-breathing exercises.

Prevent embolization
Once you detect thrombus or, in some cases, simply because
the risk of a thrombus is great, take precautions to keep the
thrombus from breaking loose. You may be able to give anticoagulants to prevent further clot formation and apply heat
locally to reduce pain and inflammation. Avoid trauma to the
threatened area and maintain a steady flow-rate. To maintain a
steady flow-rate, teach patients to avoid sudden exertion or
any sudden movements of the legs and, particularly, to avoid
holding their breath and bearing down in the Valsalva maneuver. They are especially likely to do this when having a
bowel movement or when turning in bed. As you know, the
Valsalva maneuver may cause reflex slowing of heart rate or
temporary heart block. The great danger to a patient with a
thrombus is that such straining also greatly increases intrathoracic pressure, which reduces venous return. When the
patient stops straining, release of pressure allows a sudden surge
of venous flow, which may dislodge a thrombus.

How to recognize pulmonary embolism?

The signs, symptoms, and laboratory findings depend on the size and location of the embolus.

Large embolus: Acute cor pulmonale. Acute cor pulmonale results from an embolus large enough to occlude the pulmonary artery or one of its major branches. It usually produces a clear-cut clinical picture: pulmonary hypertension coupled with decreased venous return to the left heart and thus impaired systemic circulation. At the same time, increased pressure proximal to the obstruction increases venous pressure producing neck-vein distention, increased CVP readings, and abdominal tenderness due to liver congestion. An EKG tracing taken soon after onset of symptoms may show changes characteristic of right heart strain. Atrial arrhythmias may follow distention of the right atrium; murmurs of tricuspid or pulmonic insufficiency may follow increased right ventricular volume.

The obstruction to circulation through the lungs produces profound hemodynamic effects. In addition to the inevitable hypoxia, decreased venous return to the left heart causes decreased ventricular filling. Hypotension develops, and the patient becomes pale, tachycardic, and apprehensive. Decreased coronary and cerebral perfusion appear as anginal pain and mental confusion. This clinical picture rarely calls for further diagnostic tests. (An exception: Pulmonary angiograms are needed before embolectomy.)

Medium embolus: Infarction. Pulmonary infarction (necrosis of lung tissue) may occur when an embolus occludes a medium sized artery and decreases circulation to the surrounding pulmonary parenchyma by the bronchial arteries. Systemic hypotension or pulmonary venous hypertension compromises bronchial circulation and is most likely in patients with infected, congested, or hypoventilated lungs. Pulmonary infarction is not usually fatal, and often facilitates the diagnosis of pulmonary embolism. Still, its symptoms and physical findings vary from patient to patient, so you must watch for its most prevalent findings to recognize it.

Small and medium emboli: Varying symptoms. Some small emboli produce no symptoms at all. Others can mimic a myocardial infarction, dissecting aortic aneurysm, pericarditis, congestive heart failure, pneumonia, bronchitis, and simple episodes of arrhythmias.

What are its usual symptoms? Most patients develop dyspnea and a cough. Many patients complain of feelings of apprehension

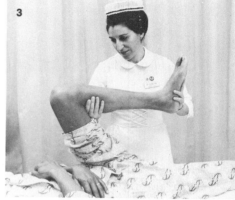

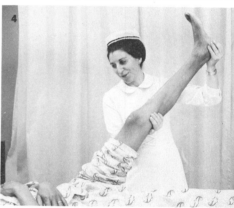

3. Move his leg slowly back toward his head as far as it will go without hurting him.

4. Straighten his knee by lifting the foot upward. Lower his leg to the starting position and repeat the exercise.

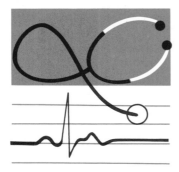

Diagnostic profile

LAB TESTS
WBC — If infarction is present, may be normal or elevated but is usually less than 15,000, with little or no increase in differential count. This helps rule out acute pneumonia in which the WBC often exceeds 15,000.
PO_2— decreased; often below 80 mm Hg. PO_2 above 80 mm Hg usually rules out pulmonary embolism.
PCO_2— below normal (34 to 46 mm Hg).

ELECTROCARDIOGRAM
Circulatory obstruction *may* cause:
 • right axis deviation
 • right bundle-branch block pattern in V_1
 • sinus tachycardia
 • tall peaked P waves (P pulmonale)
 • shifts in S-T segment and T wave directions
 • sudden onset of atrial flutter, atrial fibrillation, or other supraventricular tachycardias.

CHEST X-RAY
You may see a diaphragm elevation, pleural fluid on the affected side, and prominence of a pulmonary artery. A triangular shadow, indicating necrosis, may appear in pulmonary infarction patients. It's diagnostic.

or impending disaster. More than half have pain, usually in the chest but occasionally in the abdomen or flank. The character of the pain ranges from pleuritic to a close mimic of angina. Relatively few have hemoptysis (only 40% of emboli with infarctions). Cyanosis is rare.

Physical findings are even less specific. The combination of unexplained tachycardia, tachypnea, and fever is generally considered most characteristic of pulmonary embolism, but these same findings preexist in many patients with other pulmonary or cardiac diseases. However, four findings occur regularly in at least half of all patients: 1) an increased intensity of the pulmonic component of the second heart sound due to pulmonary hypertension (in about 80%); 2) tachypnea — more than 20 respirations per minute (in 75%); 3) pulmonary rales (in 70%); and 4) tachycardia (in 65%). Less often, patients may have an abnormal third heart sound (S_3 gallop), phlebitis, fever, and a pleural friction rub (fever and pleural friction rub are more typical of infarction than of simple embolus).

Because clinical findings are so inconclusive, the following diagnostic tests are generally ordered to confirm pulmonary embolism:
 • Lab studies, as shown on the left, usually include white blood count, erythrocyte sedimentation rate, serum enzymes, and arterial blood gases.
 • A chest X-ray rules out other pulmonary pathology.
 • A lung scan is one of the most useful confirming procedures (see page 139).
 • An EKG may distinguish between acute myocardial infarction and pulmonary embolism.
 • Pulmonary angiography is the most definitive test. Through a dye-injection technique, angiography pinpoints the exact location of an embolus in the pulmonary arterial tree.

Treatment two-fold
The treatment of acute pulmonary embolism requires support of vital functions and prevention of further emboli. Death, when it occurs, is due to circulatory failure, and 3 out of 4 such deaths occur within a few hours. In patients who survive, circulation begins to seep past the clot as pressure builds up next to it. Improvement thereafter is usually rapid.

Treatment measures include:
 • *Bedrest* is necessary to prevent further embolization, but the

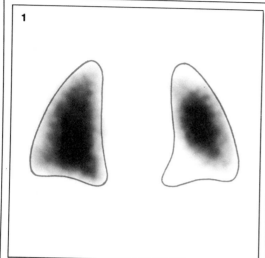

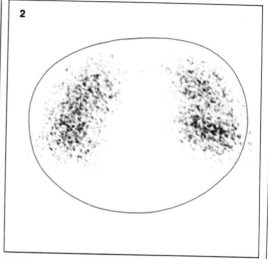

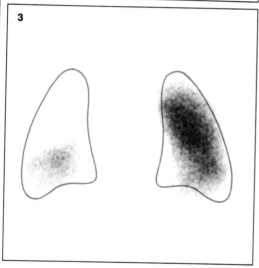

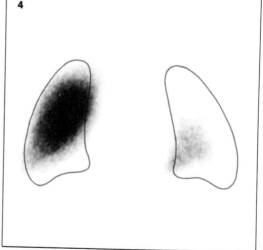

What lung scans show

Lung scans show pulmonary blood flow. Emboli too small to be picked up by angiogram can be seen on a lung scan. Blood perfusion is shown by the dark areas. Figure 1 shows a normal lung scan.

Often ordered in conjunction with the scan is an equilibrium test. For this test, the patient inhales an inert gas, such as xenon, along with oxygen for 30 seconds. The scan which photographs xenon then shows lung ventilation. Figure 2 shows a normal equilibrium.

To assess the total lung field, scans are taken from two different views. Figure 3 shows an anterior view and Figure 4 shows a posterior view. In both cases you can see that the right apical segment is incompletely perfused due to a pulmonary embolus.

nurse must be prepared to combat all the additional hazards of immobility.

- *Oxygen* is given either by mask or by cannula.
- *Vasopressors* may be used for severe circulatory failure.
- *Heparin* is given in an initial I.V. injection of 10,000 to 15,000 units. (Subcutaneous administration is rarely used because of uneven absorption with this route.) Oral anticoagulants may be started at the same time or delayed for a few days. Most patients can begin oral anticoagulants after 4 to 7 days of heparin.
- *Narcotics* are given to relieve pain and apprehension.
- *Digitalization* may begin (although at less than full digitalizing dose because myocardial ischemia can result from poor coronary artery perfusion).
- *Intravenous fluids* may be given to combat shock. If so, monitor central venous pressure.
- *Thrombolytic agents*, such as urokinase (Abbokinase) and streptokinase (Streptase), may be used to dissolve the embolus and the original thrombus.
- *Embolectomy* is considered only in patients who have profound circulatory failure or who cannot be anticoagulated.

Remember these important points about pulmonary embolisms:

1. Watch for this condition in patients recovering from surgery; patients with myocardial infarctions, cerebrovascular accidents, congestive heart failure, fractures, and burns; and elderly patients with debilitating diseases.

2. Prevent venous stasis and, in turn, a pulmonary embolism by repositioning and exercising your patient's legs, encouraging early ambulation, applying antiembolism elastic stockings, and teaching him deep-breathing exercises.

3. Keep a thrombus from breaking loose by avoiding trauma to the threatened area and by telling your patient to avoid sudden exertion, any sudden leg movements, holding his breath, and bearing down, as in Valsalva's maneuver.

4. Be aware that a PO_2 level above 80 mm Hg helps rule out pulmonary embolism as the cause of your patient's symptoms.

5. Consider calm reassurance your most important contribution to your patient's care.

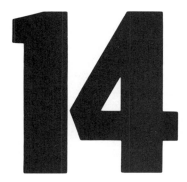

Pacemakers
Help for the faltering heart

BY MINNIE BOWEN ROSE, RN, BSN, MEd

MR. MACKENZIE WAS WORKING as a night clerk in a small hotel when he fell and couldn't get up. An ambulance brought him to the emergency room where he seemed weak and slightly confused. His heart rate was 48; his blood pressure, 169/80. He didn't seem to be in acute distress. But when an EKG strip showed third-degree atrioventricular block, Mr. Mackenzie became a candidate for artificial pacing of his heart, and was admitted for cardiac evaluation.

The number of patients with pacemakers is growing every year and, chances are, you'll work with someone like Mr. Mackenzie sooner or later. Do you know all you really should about pacemakers? How to detect failure in their mechanism? How to answer patients' questions about them and properly prepare them to live with a pacemaker? If not, you may benefit from reading this chapter.

Pacemakers are increasingly being implanted temporarily in hospitalized patients — those with transient blockage of conductive pathways from edema, ischemia from coronary artery disease or following heart surgery, or myocardial infarction. For example, after heart surgery, while the chest is still open, surgeons routinely implant pacing electrodes on the epicar-

Patients for pacing

In the early days of pacemaking, the sole indication was complete atrioventricular block leading to Stokes-Adams attacks.
Nowadays, doctors implant pacemakers for many conduction defects, ranging from complete to partial and/or intermittent AV block. Accepted indications include:
• complete AV block lasting 1 to 3 weeks or more following acute myocardial infarction
• complete AV block associated with congestive heart failure or cerebral or renal insufficiency that improves with temporary pacing
• persistent AV block following cardiac surgery
• need for prophylaxis following cardiac surgery
• incomplete AV block (Mobitz Type II or advanced second-degree block)
• symptomatic bilateral bundle branch block
• symptomatic sinus bradycardia, with or without AV block
• sinus arrest or sinoatrial block
• sick sinus syndrome
• trifascicular block
• atrial tachycardia
• need for improved cardiac output.

dium. They extend them through the chest incision and connect them to an external pacing battery box. The pacemaker is then a ready backup to be used as needed within the next few days: to control any arrhythmias that may develop after surgery; to increase the heart rate; or to improve cardiac output (if low output is due to brady- or tachyarrhythmias).

Artificial electric pacing almost always begins with a temporary transvenous pacemaker. Most implants are made through the subclavian, antecubital, external jugular, or femoral vein. A temporary pacemaker is relatively simple for the trained doctor to insert. It needs neither general anesthesia nor thoracotomy, but only a venous cutdown or percutaneous placement under local anesthesia. Its batteries are easy to replace, and the device can easily be removed when pacing is no longer needed.

Of course, temporary pacemakers have some obvious disadvantages: A disoriented patient can pull the catheter; electrodes may break, be dislodged, or perforate the ventricular wall; or the site of insertion can become infected. Then, too, the patient's constant awareness of being hooked up to external lifesaving equipment may cause him marked anxiety.

Permanent pacing

When a patient has irreversible cardiac damage with a complete block in the conduction system of the heart, he needs a permanent pacemaker. It, too, can be inserted intravenously. The difference between this and the temporary pacer is that its generator gets permanently implanted within the subcutaneous tissue of the patient's chest or abdomen.

Less often, the permanent electrodes get implanted transthoracically. The surgeon opens the chest anteriorly and sutures the electrodes into the epicardial surface of the ventricle. Then he threads the wires through a subcutaneous tunnel to the battery box, and sets them under the chest or abdominal skin. The chief drawback in this method: The patient must endure a major operation and the usual postoperative course of a thoracotomy. Problems with permanent pacemakers are relatively few. But infection at the implantation site is possible; any malfunction requires another surgical procedure.

Prepare patients for pacing

Pacemakers have saved countless lives. Yet, beyond a doubt,

the patient who has one is acutely aware of his dependence on this artificial heartbeat. Anything you can do to prepare him for it, help him get used to it, and teach him to live with it at home is a valuable service indeed. You'll usually be working with someone elderly; 70% of pacemaker patients are over 60. But some are young people, including infants born with a heart block. Men outnumber women 2 to 1.

Because the patient will surely forget some of what the surgeon tells him before the operation, it's a good idea for you to be there for the explanation. You can help him absorb it later. For example, you can tell him that the actual insertion of the device will be done through a small incision and under local anesthesia.

If he's getting a permanent pacemaker, show him a model of it and let him handle it. To minimize complications, emphasize the need for him to return to activity. According to his response to this advice, help him determine goals. Above all, help him understand that a pacemaker can return him to an active life his own heartbeat can no longer support. Try to explain all this to his family or closest relative, too, if possible while family and patient are together. Naturally they'll be worried. Remember to warn them kindly that getting through the operation successfully does not automatically guarantee recovery without complications.

It seems easier to prepare a patient for temporary pacing than for permanent pacing. Nonetheless, the short-term patient is often more apprehensive because the whole situation is so new to him. With patience and understanding, you can help him over this critical stage. You can help reduce the physiologic strain his emotions are adding to an already over-taxed heart.

After implantation
The patient will probably need bedrest for the rest of the day, and maybe for 48 hours. But after that, he should get up and walk around as soon as possible.

Resume your monitoring and run an EKG strip immediately for analysis of the pacemaker function. Check the incision site for bleeding, redness, warmth of the incision site, swelling, or pain. Expect some normal bloody drainage, but keep the skin as clean and dry as possible. Take vital signs as ordered and check for fever. Check the prescribed setting of the pacemaker, and record it in your notes. If things are going well, revise your nursing care plan to include patient-teaching requirements — especially if the patient has, or is going to have, a permanent device.

Keep the cardiac monitor going for about 24 hours to be sure the pacemaker is functioning properly and the electrodes haven't dislodged. Explain the importance of his continued monitoring meantime, and tell why you must watch his vital functions closely. Urge him to report any symptoms: faintness, hiccups, or pain. Patients usually have some pain at the operative site and need an analgesic. However, report persistent or increasing pain to the doctor. Make nursing observations frequently, and keep checking vital signs.

Watch for complications
Complications that may follow thoracic installation of the pacemaker? They primarily result from the chest surgery itself: pneumonia, atelectasis, embolism, or the like. So, the patient will need deep-breathing, intermittent positive-pressure breathing, coughing, and regular turning from side to side. These measures will help loosen bronchial secretions and keep lungs well expanded.

Certain complications may follow implantation of any kind of pacemaker. You need to recognize them promptly.

• *An electrode may break (infrequently) or be dislodged.* Then the QRS complex, which signifies contraction of the ventricles, will change contour on the cardiac monitor. The heart rate itself will noticeably slow down if pacing fails. When this happens the electrode must be repaired, replaced, or repositioned.

• *An electrode may perforate the ventricle wall.* Watch for hiccups, a sign of spasm of the upper-abdominal or lower-chest muscles stimulated by a stray electrode; you may save the patient's life. Also be alert for cardiac tamponade, in which blood in the pericardium compresses the heart. The signs of tamponade are low blood pressure, increased venous pressure, distended neck veins, increased pulse rate, decreased urinary output, cyanosis, and restlessness. If you suspect cardiac tamponade or stray electrode, notify the doctor at once: Immediate surgery is needed.

• *The pacemaker may malfunction; the heart may resist.* For the first 2 or 3 days after implantation, the heart is highly

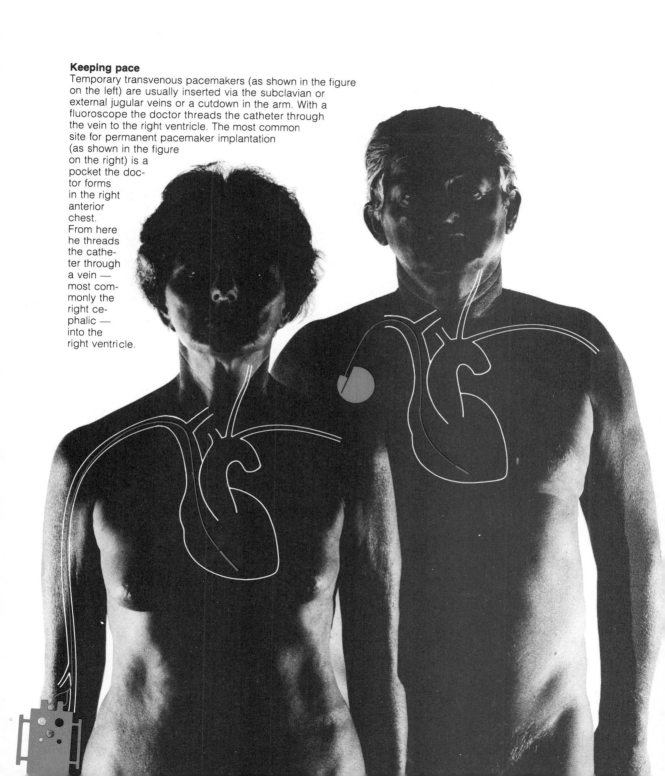

Keeping pace

Temporary transvenous pacemakers (as shown in the figure on the left) are usually inserted via the subclavian or external jugular veins or a cutdown in the arm. With a fluoroscope the doctor threads the catheter through the vein to the right ventricle. The most common site for permanent pacemaker implantation (as shown in the figure on the right) is a pocket the doctor forms in the right anterior chest. From here he threads the catheter through a vein — most commonly the right cephalic — into the right ventricle.

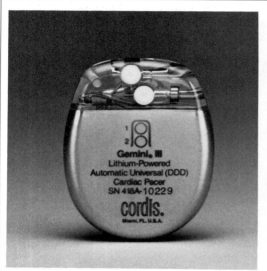

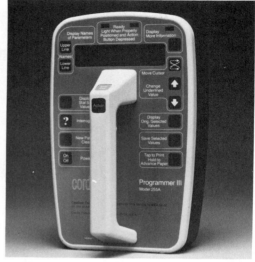

KINDS OF IMPLANTABLE PACEMAKERS

A three-letter identification code for implantable cardiac pacemakers helps you to sort out their complex characteristics. The first letter identifies the paced chamber: V stands for ventricle, A for atrium, and D for double (atrium and ventricle). The second letter identifies the sensed chamber: A or V. The third letter identifies the response mode: I for inhibited and T for triggered. The letter O means no specific comment is applicable. Possible pacemaker combinations include VOO, AOO, DOO, VVI, VVT, AAI, AAT, VAT, and DVI.

Pacemakers are commonly grouped by pacing mode.

FIXED RATE PACEMAKERS (AOO, VOO, DOO) keep a steady rate regardless of the patient's own cardiac impulses. Fixed rate pacemakers are rarely used.

QRS-INHIBITED PACEMAKER (VVI), a demand pacemaker with an inhibited response mode, prevents firing of an impulse when the pacemaker senses an R wave.

QRS-TRIGGERED PACEMAKER (VVT) fires in the absolute refractory pe-

riod when it senses the R wave. Thus, when natural cardiac rhythm is adequate, this pacemaker fires but causes no cardiac response. However, if cardiac rate falls below the pacemaker's preset rate, the artificial discharge stimulates the myocardium to contract.

ATRIAL SYNCHRONIZED PACEMAKER (VAT) uses an atrial electrode to sense normal atrial depolarization. Then, after an appropriate delay, it triggers a ventricular electrode to pace the ventricle. If the atrial rate exceeds 130 beats/minute, the pacemaker transmits every other impulse to the ventricle. If the rate falls below 60, the pacer initiates fixed pacing at 60 beats/minute.

ATRIOVENTRICULAR SEQUENTIAL PACING (DVI) imitates the normal sequence of electrical activity in the heart, maintaining cardiac output 22% higher than conventional pacemakers. It uses two separate electrodes to pace the atrium and ventricle in sequence. However, it's inhibited by ventricular activity.

Pacemakers can also be grouped according to their use.

VENTRICULAR PACEMAKERS (QRS-inhibited, QRS-triggered, and some

temporary pacemakers) are primarily (95%) used to treat sinus bradycardia. They may be permanent or temporary.

ATRIAL PACEMAKERS (AAI, AAT, and some temporary pacemakers) are used when AV conduction is intact, especially for symptomatic bradycardia and sick sinus syndrome, with or without congestive heart failure and low cardiac output. Rapid atrial pacing is helpful to end intractable supraventricular and ventricular tachyarrhythmias.

ATRIAL SYNCHRONOUS PACEMAKER (VAT and some temporary pacemakers) are commonly used when complete heart block prevents use of an atrial pacemaker or when another condition prevents ventricular pacing because the patient needs atrial contraction to maintain cardiac output.

AUTOMATIC DDD PACEMAKER (AAI + VATO + VVI), shown above left, can be programmed to sense and/or pace the atria and ventricules. This pacer allows for consistent A-V synchrony. A hand-held portable programmer (above right) permits the doctor to make adjustments in pacer modes.

QUESTIONS PACEMAKER PATIENTS ASK

What am I allowed to do now that I have a pacemaker?
Generally, anything you enjoyed before. You can even play sports, as soon as the doctor gives you permission. He'll probably have you begin by walking and then gradually increase your activity. You should even be able to swim. The only athletic restriction you must observe is to avoid body contact sports, such as football.

As to sex, you can return to whatever degree of activity you want and can tolerate.

Can I return to work?
Yes, whenever the doctor says you may. Discuss your work with him. If you're a telephone lineman, you may have to switch to less strenuous work. If you're a banker or an accountant, you should be able to resume your duties. Jobs that involve working near equipment that can disrupt pacing (such as high tension wires and electrical generators) are unsuitable.

What daily medical care must I practice? Do I have to check my pulse often?
Yes, at least once a day for 60 seconds. The nurse will show you how, and what variations mean. Have a family member learn also. Keep a daily record of your pulse rate to bring to your next checkup. If your pulse rate drops below that set by the pacemaker, notify your doctor.

The nurse will explain your medications to you and any precautions they require. Follow your doctor's orders about diet.

Take your medications as prescribed. Don't skip doses or vary the times you take them. Keep a record of what you take and when you take it, and bring this along with your pulse record to

your next checkup.

Can water hurt my pacemaker?
Don't wet the incision site until after the doctor removes the sutures. After that, however, no amount of water will hurt.

How do I care for my incision?
Be careful to keep it clean and dry. Wash the incision with mild soap and water; then dry gently.

Don't wear clothing that rubs or presses against the slight bump on your chest over the pacemaker unit. For example, a woman with a chest implant shouldn't wear tight bras. But if clothing, such as a bra strap, rubs against the incision, cover the incision with a light dressing to avoid irritation.

If you notice redness, discharge, or pain over the implant, report it to your doctor.

What else should I watch for?
Report any dizziness, vertigo, shortness of breath, unwarranted fatigue, prolonged hiccups, nausea, vomiting, diarrhea, or a very fast or very slow heart rate.

Can I travel?
Yes, you can resume driving a car after about a month, but avoid lengthy travel of any kind for at least 3 months after implant and then again during the later stages of battery life. Tell your doctor of your plans before you travel, and carry a list of doctors and hospitals in the appropriate locales to use if needed.

Pacemaker patients should always carry an ID card that gives a medical summary, the kind of pacemaker they have, its rate, and their doctor's name, address, and telephone number.

May I fly in a plane?
Yes, but if you must pass

through an airport metal detector, alert the authorities that you have a pacemaker since the metal in it may set off an alarm.

Can electrical equipment harm me?
In general, no. Household appliances, if properly grounded, can't disrupt your pacemaker. But avoid using an electric shaver directly over the implanted unit. Also avoid standing or leaning over electric motors or gasoline engines. They can cause palpitations or an irregular heart rate and make you feel faint. But this will stop if you leave the area. For the same reasons, stay well out of the high-voltage electric fields that emanate from overhead utility transmission lines.

If you're having your teeth fixed or must have surgery, tell your dentist or surgeon that you have a pacemaker. You might need to take a prophylactic antibiotic to prevent any bloodborne infections. Consult your cardiologist before undergoing any medical procedure that involves electricity.

How long will my pacemaker last?
Some last as long as 9 to 10 years.

What happens if it stops working?
Don't lose sleep over this! Your pacemaker clinic will replace the unit before it stops. Changing batteries involves only a simple procedure. But if the pacemaker does stop, the heart will slow to its former rate.

Have regular checkups, not because your pacemaker may fail but because your needs may change and your pacemaker may need resetting.

Pacemaker tips

- Explain to the patient why the procedure is necessary and how it will be performed.
- Show the patient a pacemaker; explain how it works.
- Watch him carefully after insertion to verify that the pacemaker is functioning properly and effectively.
- Watch for loss of capture, competition, signs of perforation, thrombophlebitis, or skin infection.
- Tell the patient and his family at what rate his pacemaker is set.

TEMPORARY PACEMAKER
- After the electrode has been introduced, gradually turn the energy control dial clockwise until you note a QRS complex with each stimulus. This is the patient's threshold level (usually about 1.5 milliamperes). As a safety precaution, this number is usually doubled to assure continued pacing.
- If loss of capture occurs:

(continued, opposite page)

sensitive to the electrode within it. Especially during that time, look for any disturbance in cardiac rhythm, such as PVCs and runs of ventricular tachycardia; signs of pacemaker failure, changing of rate, failure to capture, and return of symptoms such as syncope; or need to adjust the pacing rate. In some hospitals, you may be allowed to adjust the rate and sensitivity on an external power generator as necessary. In others, you can only monitor and report changes.

If the monitor shows premature ventricular extrasystoles or other ectopic activity, the patient may need immediate treatment with: antiarrhythmic drugs, restoration of normal potassium balance, or an increase in the pacing rate.

- *Watch for infection.* Contamination of the equipment or wound during the procedure or afterward can produce thrombophlebitis, septicemia, or endocarditis. You can help avoid these by using a rigorously aseptic technique in preparing the site, and later by watching the patient for any signs of infection.
- *Keep the extremity mobile.* When a temporary pacemaker is inserted in the antecubital vein, the patient's elbow must, of course, be immobilized to protect the site of insertion. Nevertheless, the patient needs to wiggle his fingers freely. He needs some range-of-motion exercises for his shoulder to avoid stiffness. Encourage every patient with permanent pacemakers in the upper-outer chest wall to exercise the arm on that side before and after the implantation. However, such exercises, any over-the-head motion of the arms, or any turning on the side should not begin for 24 to 72 hours after implantation (to avoid dislodgement of the catheter tip).

Troubleshooting the pacemaker

Suspect malfunction when you see symptoms of heart block return — such as syncope, slow pulse, and convulsions. Also suspect it when you see premature beats or changes in rhythm.

In many hospitals, an EKG technician will check a patient's temporary pacemaker daily. But you can check its function yourself. It's simple. With a stethoscope, listen to the patient's apical pulse and watch the sense-pace dial (on a temporary pulse generator). Use the apical pulse because the radial pulse is far enough away from the heart that the lag time between heartbeat and pulse is too great, particularly at faster rates. Whenever you suspect pacemaker malfunction, check the patient's pulse rate, blood pressure, level of consciousness, and respiratory status. If the apical rate has dropped too much, perfusion may be inadequate, and the patient may be at risk for cardiac arrest.

Firing: If the sense-pace dial on a temporary pacemaker generator shows the pacer has fired, and a split-second later you hear the pulse, you know the pacer is firing and capturing properly. If the sense-pace is *not* registering, you know the pacemaker has stopped firing. The usual cause: Someone inadvertently turned off the power switch. Other causes are malfunctioning electronic circuitry and dead batteries in the pulse generator. So, make sure the power switch is on, check all connections, and change the battery in the pulse generator. If firing doesn't resume, replace the pulse generator.

Capturing: If the sense-pace dial shows firing, but you hear no corresponding apical pulse, you know the pacemaker is not capturing. Suspect loss of capture when the patient's heart rate is less than the rate set on the pulse generator. Loss of capture usually results from displacement of the catheter tip. The tip is often wedged behind the trabeculae in the wall near the apex of the right ventricle. The tip may dislodge and float freely in the right ventricle, may advance in the right ventricle, may advance into the pulmonary artery, or may retract into the right atrium. Rarely the tip will perforate the wall of the ventricle and lodge outside the heart. This may cause the pacemaker to capture the diaphragm (which gives the patient hiccups at the rate set on the pulse generator, ventricular tachycardia, or ventricular fibrillation).

Another cause of loss of capture: ischemia of the myocardium or fibrosis near the tip. Ischemic tissue has a higher threshold and, so, needs more energy to depolarize the myocardium and produce a contraction. Some rarer causes: The negative terminal of the pulse generator becomes disconnected from the distal wire of the pacing catheter; or the power cable or catheter breaks.

What to do about loss of capture? Turn the patient on his left side, which may let the catheter fall back in contact with the right ventricle wall. Turn up the setting of the output dial. If ischemic myocardium is the cause, the increased amperage may compensate for it.

Sensing: If the patient's apical pulse is higher than the rate set on the pulse generator, but the sense-pace dial shows

change the patient's position, the battery, or the pacemaker unit. Notify the doctor.
- When discontinuing the pacemaker, turn the rate down *gradually* to avoid causing asystole.

PERMANENT PACEMAKER
- Teach the patient and family how to count and record his pulse daily.
- Explain the signs of battery failure: change in pacing rate, dizziness, Stokes-Adams attacks, dyspnea, or increased weight gain.
- Have the patient watch for signs of infection or skin breakdown.
- Tell him when to notify the doctor: when pulse rate changes; symptoms recur; he has signs of infection; or has suffered a blow that may have damaged his pacemaker.
- Make sure the patient understands the necessity of follow-up care at regular intervals.

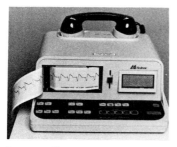

Let your fingers do the walking
Reassure your patient that checking pacemaker function is as easy as picking up the phone. For example, the Medtronic pacemaker uses a Medtronic Model 9408 TeleTrace Transmitter to telephone an EKG signal to the doctor's office or clinic.

Explain to your patient that at an appointed time he'll call a predetermined phone number. Then, he'll rest a small rectangular transmitter against his bare chest and put the telephone's mouthpiece against the transmitter's speaker. The transmitter will detect electrical signals generated by the patient's pacemaker and convert them to sound waves. The telephone receiver will then send these sound waves to a receiver in the office or clinic (see photo above), which will convert them to an EKG readout strip. By examining the strip, the doctor will be able evaluate pacemaker function.

continuous firing at the lower rate, the pacer is not sensing the patient's own heart rate. The pacer should never fire when the patient's own rate consistently exceeds the pacer's set rate. In this situation, called competition, the pacer is competing with the patient's own pacemaker for control of his heart instead of assisting it. This causes an irregular heart rhythm. Competition is dangerous because it may cause ventricular fibrillation if the pacer fires during the myocardium's recovery or repolarization phase at the top of the T wave.

What causes it? Most likely, the catheter tip has moved so that the sensing electrode doesn't receive a strong enough signal from the patient's myocardium. Indeed, the tip may be displaced so much that both sensing and capture are lost. Again, other causes include broken or disconnected wiring. What to do? Turn the patient on his left side, which may move the pacing catheter back into place. Check the demand dial to make sure it is in the full demand position. If neither of these procedures restores proper function, and if the patient's own rate is adequate to maintain circulation, follow your hospital's policy. Some hospitals may want you to turn the pacemaker off to prevent ventricular fibrillation and call the doctor at once to reposition the catheter.

Patient teaching vital
When a temporary pacemaker is stopped, be sure that the patient does not feel any anxiety about its being discontinued. If he does, reassure him. When a patient with a temporary pacemaker is to get a permanent one, explain how he will live with his new equipment. Usually, the interval between temporary and permanent implantations is long enough to allow a relaxed period of preparation.

Remember these important points about pacemakers:
1. Consider a patient with a conduction defect, either a complete or second-degree type II AV block, a possible pacemaker candidate.
2. Watch for signs of pacemaker complications: a broken or dislodged electrode (loss of capture), electrode perforation of the ventricular wall (hiccups or cardiac tamponade), and malfunction (disturbances in heart rhythm).
3. Suspect loss of capture when the patient's heart rate is less than the rate set on the pulse generator.

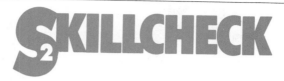

SKILLCHECK

1. How does hypertension predispose to coronary artery disease?

2. Why do patients with angina frequently experience pain in the left shoulder and arm?

3. Which of the following patients is most at risk for a pulmonary embolus: a 42-year-old male in CCU, 3 days postmyocardial infarction; a 16-year-old male 6 days after knee surgery; a 31-year-old obese primipara, 5 days postCaesarean section; a 28-year-old male immobilized in traction for 36 days following a motorcycle accident.

4. Martha is a 56-year-old woman who has been hospitalized for a fractured pelvis for the past 24 days. You notice that her respirations have suddenly gone from 16/min. to 32/min., although her color is unchanged. She is complaining of chest pain and looks very apprehensive. Her blood pressure is unchanged, but her pulse is 116/min. regular and her temperature is 100.4° F. (38° C.). She had rales in both bases but no S_3 or S_4. What's the most likely explanation for her symptoms? What should you do?

5. John is a 38-year-old black male who comes to your clinic because of fatigue and early morning headaches. On ophthalmoscopy you notice soft exudates, hemorrhages, and papilledema. What condition do these findings suggest and what is John's probable prognosis?

6. The most specific serum enzyme study used to diagnose an AMI is: CPK, CPK-MB, SGOT, or LDH?

7. Which of these EKG findings is *not* typical of an AMI: Deep Q waves, S-T elevation, S-T depression, or T wave inversion?

8. How does Inderal reduce myocardial oxygen consumption?

9. Tom Beal has just been admitted to your unit to "Rule out AMI." He had chest pain at home 4 hours ago, received morphine sulfate, 4 mg I.V., in the E.D., and is now complaining of nausea and is vomiting. What is happening? What should you watch for?

10. On auscultation you notice that Tom's heart sounds are abnormal: There are 3 sounds instead of 2. What does this mean? Should you call his doctor?

11. Tom is asking for something for pain. Should you give the medication (Demerol 75 mg.) I.M. or I.V.?

12. John Anderson is a patient on your unit who is 6 days post MI. He's been recovering uneventfully. When you bring in his evening medication you find him unresponsive. His vital signs are: BP 90/60, P 154/min., R 32/min. You notice that his BP varies 15 mm Hg with respiration (pulsus paradoxus). He is lying at a 45° angle but his neck veins are distended to 20 cm. What has happened?

(Answers on page 171)

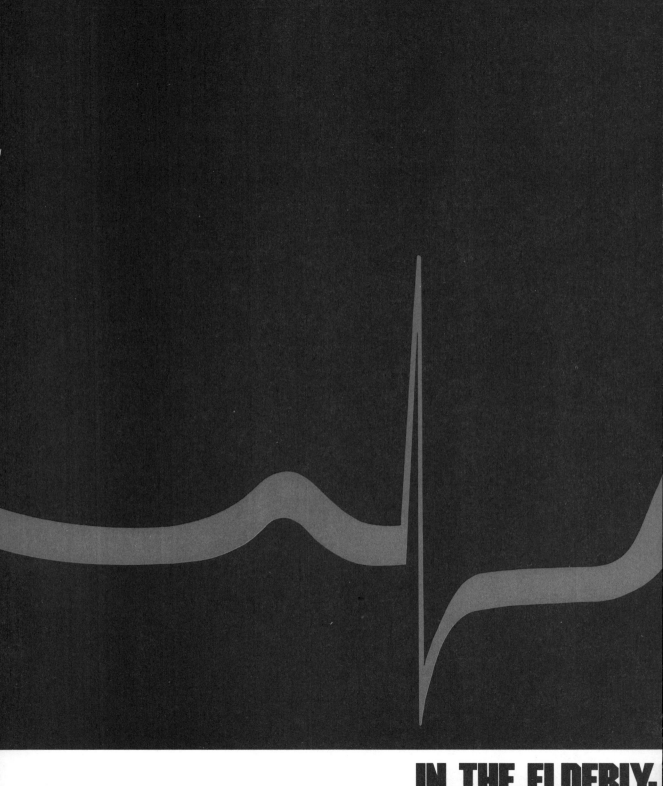

IN THE ELDERLY:

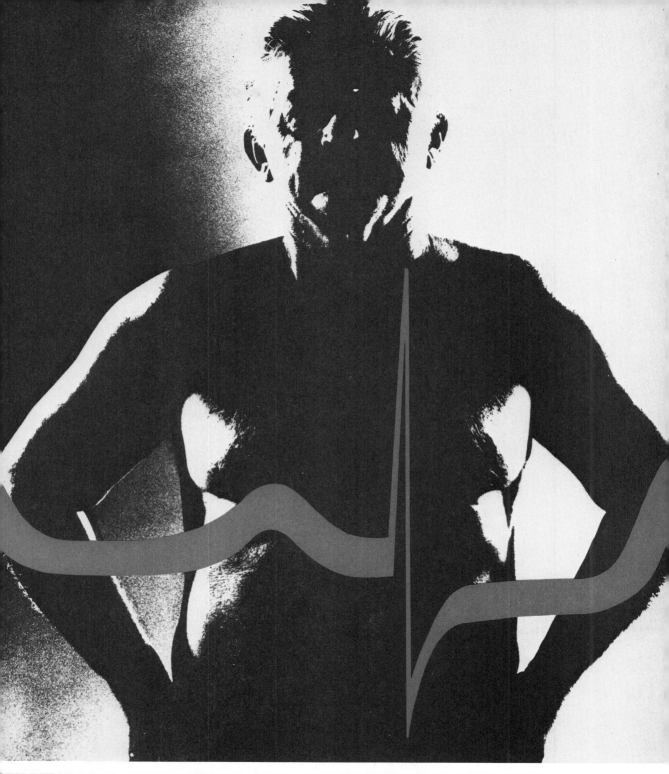

EXPECT VASCULAR DETERIORATION

What can the soles of your patient's feet tell
you about arterial insufficiency?

If your patient has venous insufficiency,
what signs and symptoms would
you expect to find?

What relatively new drug is being used
to treat Raynaud's disease?

What are the signs of aneurysm rupture?

What nursing actions can you take to prevent
your patient from developing adult
respiratory distress syndrome following an
aneurysm resection?

If your patient has an aneurysm that is less
than 6 cm, what diagnostic tests will help
monitor the size of the aneurysm?

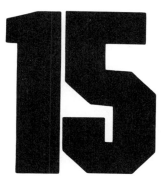

Peripheral Vascular Disease
Cause of leg pain

BY IDABELLE REAM, RN

UNLESS YOUR NURSING CARE involves only the very young, you probably often hear patients complain of aching legs. Elderly patients are especially likely to complain of cramps, fullness, and aching in the legs. Do you dismiss such complaints lightly? Or do you consider them a likely sign of peripheral vascular disease...of arterial or venous insufficiency? Both can lead to progressive suffering and disability unless they're promptly and correctly managed.

Peripheral vascular disease can be arterial, venous, or both, so you need to know the differences between them. Let's look at *arterial* disease first.

Peripheral arterial disease (arteriosclerosis is most common) causes pain in one or both legs. It forces the patient to stop walking until the pain goes away. He'll usually describe the pain as sharp — like a stabbing knife or a vise squeezing the leg. Or he may describe a feeling of unusual tiredness in one leg as he walks. Such a feeling is apt to be brought on by some change in his pattern of activity; for example, a new job that requires more walking than before. This new exertion calls attention to a condition that may have existed for years.

Peripheral arterial disease: What patients need to know

Peripheral arterial disease causes the walls of large and medium-sized peripheral arteries to thicken, harden, and lose their elasticity. As the lumen narrows, the blood flow decreases and blood clots may form. When collateral circulation cannot compensate for the block, ischemia results. The patient with arteriosclerosis, age 50 or older, will feel a vicelike pain during exercise, distal to the blockage. In advanced cases, pain may occur even during rest.

Have your patients with arteriosclerosis follow this checklist of do's and don'ts:

DO:
• Stop smoking.
• Wash feet daily and wear clean, well-fitting socks.
• Trim nails straight across but not too closely.
• Clean small cuts carefully with mild soap and water, and protect from further injury.
• Call the doctor to report any persistent leg problem.

DON'T:
• Don't go barefoot.
• Don't let your legs become extremely cold.
• Don't wear clothes that constrict your legs or feet.
• Don't let your legs get sunburned.
• Don't cut or file corns or calluses. Don't use chemical corn and callus remedies.
• Don't put a hot water bottle, heat lamp, or heating pad directly on the affected area. Instead, put the heat on the lower back or abdomen. This will warm the legs in about 15 minutes.

So your assessment should include specific questions such as, "Do your legs hurt you while you're walking?" or "Do you ever have any sharp pain in your legs?" Also ask how long such pain usually lasts. In patients with arterial insufficiency, leg pain induced by walking subsides quickly if the patient stands still for a few minutes. But if the pain persists for more than a few minutes after resting, or if it forces the patient to sit down or elevate his leg to relieve the pain, he may have some other disease. Possibilities: neuropathy or osteoarthritis. Incidentally, remember to ask elderly patients about leg pain even if they don't complain of it; many consider such pain normal at their age and not worth mentioning.

As arteriosclerosis progresses and ischemia becomes severe, the patient experiences pain even *without* exercising. He is apt to feel the pain first in the toes, heel, and dorsum of his foot. He'll probably describe such pain as a severe throbbing or ache that wakes him up after he's been in bed several hours. The pain may be increased by cold or elevation of the affected foot. For relief, he may have to rub his foot, hang it over the edge of the bed, or walk around the room.

A sensation of burning or cold often accompanies the pain of advanced arteriosclerosis. This may also be a sign of diabetic or alcoholic neuropathy. But with arteriosclerosis you'll be able to feel the cold yourself — and probably notice a diminished or absent pulse as well. With neuropathy, the foot feels warm and distal pulses are usually good.

How bad is it?

The patient's description of his leg problems can tell you the severity of arterial occlusion. If he says he can walk only about one city block without rest, he must have significant occlusion with little collateral circulation. A patient with only mild disease can walk three times as far.

To further gauge the degree of insufficiency, ask the patient to lie on his back. Taking his heels in the palm of your hand, raise both legs about 2 feet above the bed for about a minute. Then look for color changes in the skin of both feet and legs, particularly on the soles. (With dark-skinned patients, look at the soles and plantar surface of the toes.) If circulation is good, the normal pink color will diminish only slightly. If not, pallor will develop, according to the degree of occlusion. If ischemia is severe, the entire leg may become pale.

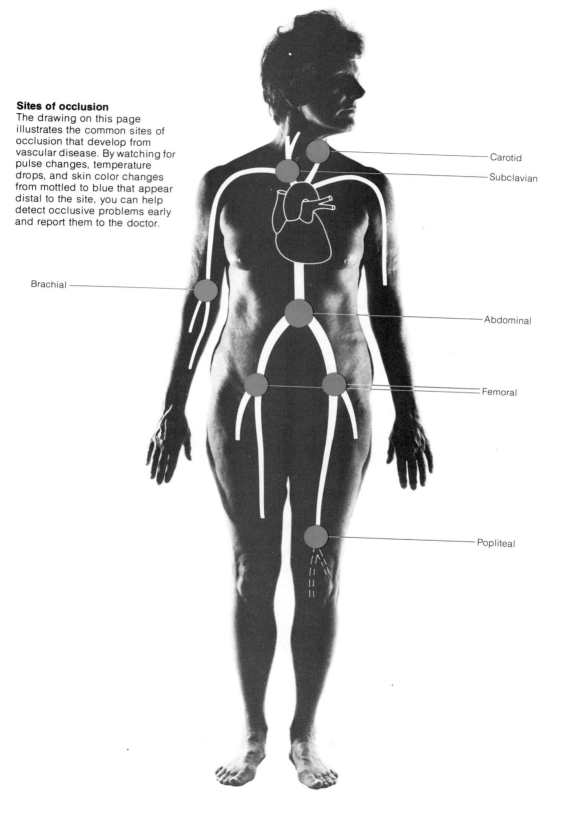

Sites of occlusion
The drawing on this page illustrates the common sites of occlusion that develop from vascular disease. By watching for pulse changes, temperature drops, and skin color changes from mottled to blue that appear distal to the site, you can help detect occlusive problems early and report them to the doctor.

Carotid

Subclavian

Brachial

Abdominal

Femoral

Popliteal

Varicose veins: What patients need to know

Varicose veins — dilated superficial leg veins — are believed to result from man's upright stance: The condition has never been found in quadrupeds.

Varicosities result from defects in the venous valves, which normally prevent retrograde blood flow. First, the proximal valves in the legs fail, increasing the column of blood that must be supported by the distal veins. The increased hydrostatic pressure distends the veins, giving them their characteristic knotlike appearance. The increased pressure may cause the capillaries to rupture, producing petechiae.

Exercise "pumps" the blood through the veins and prevents pooling. Thus the venous pressure is much lower in an active person.

To help alleviate the swelling and discomfort of varicose veins, advise your patients to:

• Avoid prolonged sitting or standing. If you must remain seated, elevate your legs whenever possible. On long car trips, stop hourly for a brief walk. If you must stand for a long time, exercise legs by periodically rising on tiptoes and shifting weight from foot to foot.

• Take a long walk daily — up to 2 miles if possible — wearing elastic bandages or stockings. Use stairs instead of elevators. Swim whenever possible.

• Never wear anything that constricts circulation such as garters or knee stockings.

• Elevate legs above heart level for an hour a day.

• Protect your legs from injury.

• Maintain a diet to prevent obesity.

If you notice pallor in *both* legs, chances are the patient has an aortoiliac block or bilateral arterial blocks in both legs. You can confirm this by having him sit up quickly and dangle his legs over the edge of the bed. The time required for color to return to the feet indicates arterial patency. With normal circulation, color returns to the feet in 10 seconds or less and superficial veins fill in 10 to 15 seconds. With significant blockage, color returns after 40 to 60 seconds; with severe blockage, after 1 to 2 minutes.

Doppler ultrasonography identifies reduced blood flow to a specific area and arterial wall thickening. However, some patients may need angiography to evaluate the need for surgery. Usual indications are:

• severe intermittent claudication that handicaps the patient physically, economically, or socially

• a sudden decrease in claudication distance

• skin changes caused by severe arterial insufficiency (including ulcers).

Preventing progression

Arterial insufficiency is not reversible, but the patient — with your guidance — can do much to prevent progression of the disease to avoid complications that might require surgery, to reduce pain, and to increase his endurance.

According to some authorities, more than a third of the amputations due to complications of arteriosclerosis result directly or indirectly from chemical, mechanical, or thermal injury. This means the patient must learn to take continuing meticulous care of his legs and know how to improve circulation. He must learn to...

• *stop smoking.* This is most important! Tobacco contains powerful vasoconstrictors that further decrease circulation and often increase pain.

• *avoid injury.* The ischemic limb is at high risk for bacterial infections, which may start with the tiniest break in the skin. "Babying" the affected leg must become second nature. (See page 156 for some do's and don'ts that will help.)

• *develop collateral circulation.* Walking is the best way to increase collateral circulation and claudication distance. Instruct the patient to walk at least 30 minutes two or three times daily. He can rest during the walk, but not the instant he begins to feel discomfort. He should walk until pain forces him to stop. When the pain goes away, he should resume walking.

Some patients become discouraged because, at first, their claudication distance decreases rather than increases. Assure them that this is common. The distance they can walk will depend on various things: temperature, walking surface, grade, and others. Nevertheless, if they persist, they will soon be walking twice as far as before without needing to rest.

Recognizing venous disorders
Some patients who complain of leg pain and fatigue may have venous insufficiency rather than arterial. The usual clues to venous involvement are:
- swollen superficial veins
- a full or tight feeling in the affected leg or legs
- leg cramps at night
- early fatigue of the leg
- leg pain during the menstrual period
- nodules or ropelike formations palpable in the legs
- swollen calves or thighs.

Certain management techniques for varicose veins are contraindicated for arterial insufficiency. So be sure these two disorders don't coexist before suggesting treatments. They often do, especially in elderly and diabetic patients. Here again, taking a good history will help. What's the most telling difference? Walking relieves venous symptoms; but it brings on claudication in patients with arterial insufficiency.

Surgery is now largely outmoded for treatment of varicosities, particularly primary (superficial) ones. Phlebography provides the best way to distinguish between primary varicosities (involving superficial veins only) and secondary varicosities (involving deep veins — deep thrombophlebitis). But other clues may help too. If the patient's history shows that the condition has developed slowly (over several years) and he has led a fairly active life, chances are that deep veins are involved. If the patient has led a sedentary life recently, or has work that requires prolonged standing on his feet (such as a waitress or sales clerk), chances favor superficial vein involvement. A family history of varicose veins also suggests superficial varicosity.

Managing mild varicosities
Uncomplicated cases of varicose veins can be managed well

SUPERFICIAL VS. DEEP THROMBOPHLEBITIS

Forming a thrombus

A century ago, a German pathologist named Rudolf Virchow identified the conditions that predispose to thrombus formation: hypercoagulability of the blood, alterations in the integrity of blood vessel walls, and venous stasis.

Hypercoagulability of the blood is associated with:
- pregnancy
- use of oral contraceptives (especially estrogen)
- postoperative states
- fever
- sickle cell anemia
- certain malignancies (especially of the pancreas)
- polycythemia vera
- abnormal "stickiness" of the platelets
- myocardial infarction.

Unfortunately, little can be done to prevent hypercoagulability other than to teach patients who take anticoagulants not to discontinue them without a doctor's supervision.

Changes in the vessel wall may result from:
- trauma
- peripheral vascular disease
- degenerative diseases
- vein distention (as of the uterine vein during pregnancy)
- pooling of the blood (as happens when the body holds one position too long).

Venous stasis results from clots caused by:
- obesity
- congestive heart failure
- arrhythmias (atrial fibrillation can cause thrombus formation in the right atrium)
- long-term immobility.

Researchers have identified the population most likely to develop a thrombus:
- women, particularly the obese
- people with a history of venous thrombosis

- people whose occupations require prolonged sitting or standing
- patients on bed rest
- postop patients
- the elderly.

Know the differences between superficial and deep thrombophlebitis so you can make a rapid, accurate assessment. Since these two conditions require different treatments, learn how to recognize the clinical distinctions and how to help the patient implement his care.

Superficial

SYMPTOMS: *Aching and swelling* usually localized into a "knot" or "bump." You can usually palpate a firm mass along the course of a superficial vein. Although this condition accompanies more symptoms than deep thrombosis, it's actually less dangerous because there's less chance of embolization.

Differential diagnosis

Insect bites (Check for history of exposure, itching, and locations away from known course of superficial vein.)
Cellulitis and abscesses (marked tenderness and peau d'orange appearance)
Subcutaneous hematoma (history of trauma, location)

USUAL LOCATION
Leg or arm. Often above or below a palpable varicose vein.

TREATMENT
Symptomatic relief for duration of symptoms, usually 2 to 3 days. Hot baths or compresses, elastic support (antiembolism) stockings. Avoidance of stasis: Walk or elevate legs. Administration of anti-inflammatory drugs, such as phenylbutazone (Butazolidin).

Deep

SYMPTOMS: *Pain* varying in degree from severe cramping to a feeling of heaviness. The patient's leg will usually feel tender. *Swelling*, the most reliable sign, may be detected only with careful bilateral measurements. (Some experts recommend that all surgery patients be measured pre- and postoperatively at the thigh, calf, and ankle to detect phlebothrombosis. This "silent" thrombosis often goes unrecognized before embolization, simply because no inflammation of the vein wall is involved.) *Homans' sign* — calf pain during dorsiflexion of the foot may be present but is not reliable. *Ramirez test* — Have patient flex his knee. Calf pain is a positive sign when you inflate a BP cuff above the knee to 40 mm Hg.

Differential diagnosis

Muscle tear (Check for history of trauma, sharp pain on exertion, ecchymosis over calf and below malleoli.)
Knee joint effusion (ballottement of patella)
Cellulitis (leukocytosis, high fever, erythema)

USUAL LOCATION
Calf vein is most common. Forty percent of patients develop thrombi bilaterally.
Femoral vein, frequently in combination with calf vein.
Iliofemoral thrombus: iliac and femoral veins.
Less common: pelvic vein and upper extremities.

TREATMENT
Prevention of emboli; bed rest and elevation of involved extremity; anticoagulation; surgical thrombectomy may be necessary if thrombus occludes a major vein.

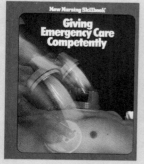
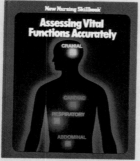
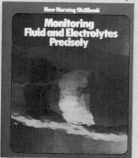
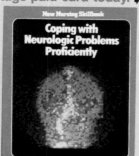
Discover how quickly and easily you can now stay abreast of the latest equipment and procedures!

Reflecting the modern, expanded role of today's nurse, each NEW NURSING SKILLBOOK offers clear instruction on how—and why—to perform current clinical procedures. You'll...

- Discover that the universal antidote for poison treatment has been proven ineffective and its use may be dangerous; learn the new poison treatment that has replaced the universal antidote.

- Learn how to avoid assessment pitfalls. For example, if you're taking only one blood pressure reading, you may be missing valuable assessment data.

- Gain insight into new techniques to relieve your patient's pain; for example, by stimulating a painful area's counterpart, you can relieve your patient's pain.

- Learn what to teach your patient about administering total parenteral nutrition at home.

- Know when to suspect an elevated central venous pressure (CVP); learn how to check quickly for an elevated CVP.

- Update your knowledge of the latest cancer chemotherapy techniques; learn how to make chemotherapy more effective with fewer side effects.

- Learn how the new calcium channel blockers help control angina; understand why assessing these drugs' effects properly is so important.

- Know why an emphysema patient should *not* receive Blocadren; understand which drugs can be administered to reverse this drug's beta-blocking effects.

- Learn about the positive emission tomography scanner and how it can help predict which stroke patients will benefit from surgery.

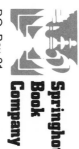
Get to know the NEW NURSING SKILLBOOK series. Examine your first—and every volume—free before you buy.

- Coping With Neurologic Problems Proficiently
- Managing Diabetics Properly
- Monitoring Fluid and Electrolytes Precisely
- Giving Cardiovascular Drugs Safely
- Assessing Vital Functions Accurately
- Nursing Critically Ill Patients Confidently
- Giving Emergency Care Competently
- Reading EKGs Correctly
- Combatting Cardiovascular Diseases Skillfully
- Dealing with Death and Dying

Each NEW NURSING SKILLBOOK gives you ● skillchecks ● complete indexing ● easy-to-follow text that makes everything plain ● clear illustrations ● a quality hardcover binding.

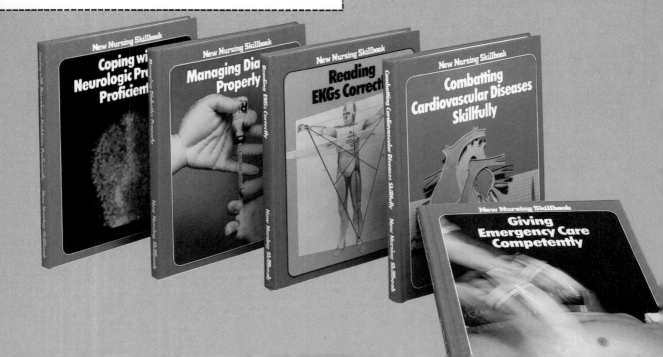

with elastic stockings and bandages. By pressing in on the legs, the elastic counteracts swelling and supports the vein walls, aiding blood-flow to the heart. Some patients prefer Ace bandages, because they can concentrate the most support to a small area where it's needed most. Whether they use stockings or bandages, patients should put them on before getting out of bed (before the leg has a chance to swell). And they should take them off before retiring, unless the doctor prescribes their nighttime use.

Not surprisingly, many patients, particularly young women, hate to wear support hose. Luckily, many of them can get adequate support from medium-weight elastic pantyhose and still be fashionable. In fact, patients with mild varicose veins can even wear standard hosiery for a few hours during social occasions without ill effects.

Patients disturbed by "spider veins" (telangiectases) can hide them easily with special cosmetics made to hide severe blemishes. Certainly, cosmetics are safer than treatment with injections of sclerosing agents. Such injections are generally only temporarily effective anyway and may lead to complications.

Dealing with stasis complications

Stasis dermatitis, induration, and ulcers sometimes result from chronic venous insufficiency. Dermatitis and induration usually heal with simple treatments: local applications of warm, moist dressings and nonirritating ointments and creams; bed rest; and elevation of the legs. Stasis ulcers are usually more serious. Before treating stasis ulcers, you must be sure that they are indeed stasis and not ischemic. This distinction is vital for patients with both arterial and venous insufficiency. Such patients need special consideration. With them, you must maintain a delicate balance — constraining the venous circulation without disrupting the arterial. That's difficult but possible.

Edema indicates the need for elastic support, but not too much. The stocking should be a lightweight type. Or, in many cases, a 4 to 6 inch elastic bandage will work better because it can be wrapped more loosely. Whatever support is selected, the patient should remove it at the first sign of any pain, then reapply it after a rest period. Sometimes, cutting the top and toe from an elastic stocking will provide the support needed

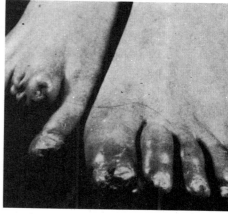

Two ischemic conditions
Two vascular diseases, Raynaud's disease and Buerger's disease, may cause ischemia, from cyanosis to gangrene.

Raynaud's disease, an idiopathic hypersensitivity to cold, affects the hands more than the feet and women more than men. Attacks may be reversible, or irreversible, involving necrosis, atrophy of the nails, and osteoporosis of the fingers and toes.

Raynaud's disease can be treated symptomatically or, in severe cases, with sympathectomy. Currently, nifedipine — a calcium channel blocker — is being used to treat Raynaud's disease.

Buerger's disease (thromboangiitis obliterans, pictured above), nonatheromatous lesions of small arteries, veins, and nerves, affects the lower extremities predominantly. The involved part suffers cold, postural color changes, pain, superficial migratory phlebitis, arteriolar spasms, and even gangrene. Doctors treat the disease symptomatically.

Patients with Buerger's or Raynaud's disease who stop smoking relieve the vasoconstriction that smoking produces.

Treating stasis ulcers
Venous insufficiency can cause painless stasis ulcers on the medial aspect of the leg. Most will require bed rest. Small ulcers can be treated by compression with an Unna boot bandage.

A stasis ulcer should be treated with povidone-iodine solution and mild topical antibiotics, if infected, and then covered with sterile dressing. The bandage must be changed daily and kept dry. To keep clean the patient should take sponge baths. If pain or seepage develops, the dressing should be changed immediately.

Stasis ulcers heal in 6 to 12 weeks. After the compression treatment, the patient should wear elastic stockings to prevent recurrence.

without restricting arterial flow. A patient who has edema and stasis symptoms, or one who's recovering from thrombophlebitis, probably needs a tailor-made heavyweight support stocking. You should examine the fit of such elastic stockings to ensure the right degree of support.

A patient with both venous and arterial insufficiency should sleep on a level bed. That is because elevating the feet will reduce edema but will also reduce arterial flow; elevating the head will increase arterial flow but also increase edema. Even better than a level bed is an *oscillating* bed, if available. Its gradual rocking reduces edema without impairing arterial circulation.

Counsel lifelong care

Once they develop, peripheral vascular diseases are usually chronic. Thus, the most important service you can offer these patients is this: Convince them of the need to continue special management after their immediate problem has been cleared up. For example, they should maintain a regular exercise program. Many elderly patients are all too willing to accept discomfort and disability as the inevitable price of growing old. However, if they remain conscientious about their leg care, they can look forward to steadily increased endurance and mobility. They can thereby maintain freedom and self-sufficiency.

Remember these important points about peripheral vascular disease:
1. Help control the progression of arteriosclerosis by advising your patient to stop smoking (nicotine is a vasoconstrictor).
2. Gauge the degree of arterial occlusion by assessing the patient's legs and feet, particularly the soles, for color changes.
3. Suspect venous insufficiency when your patient complains of swollen superficial veins, a full or tight feeling in the affected leg or legs, leg cramps at night, leg pain during the menstrual period, palpable nodules in the legs, or swollen calves or thighs.
4. Manage mild varicosities by applying elastic stockings and bandages.
5. Be aware that the calcium channel blocker nifedipine is providing relief for patients with Raynaud's disease.

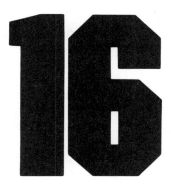

16

Aneurysm
Potentially fatal defect

BY GAIL D'ONOFRIO LONG, RN, MS

IF YOU MUST CARE for an aneurysm patient, you may have trouble on your hands. First of all, given the typical age group of such patients (60 to 70), you must be on the lookout for signs of pulmonary impairment and even cerebral complications of atherosclerosis. Then, because the surgical repair of the condition requires a massive incision — from xiphoid to pubis — the patient can easily bleed and leak fluid. Here's what to expect in (and do for) such a patient.

Chances are — by four to one — that your patient with an abdominal aortic aneurysm (AAA) will be a man like Sidney Rosoff, a 63-year-old math teacher with atherosclerosis. Mr. Rosoff's annual physical exam revealed a pulsatile mass in the midabdominal region. When questioned, the only symptom he admitted was a dull epigastric pain and a feeling of fullness after meals. But he'd assumed it was indigestion.

Mr. Rosoff's case is not unusual. In fact, more than half the people with an aneurysm have no symptoms. When symptoms do occur, they arise from the aneurysm's pressure on surrounding structures, from its stretching of the mesenteric root, or from slow leakage of blood causing retroperitoneal pressure.

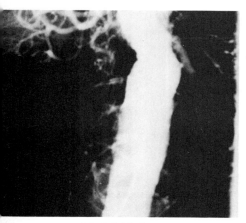

A baleful bulge
This arteriogram shows an abdominal aortic aneurysm before surgery. The aneurysm does not extend to the renal arteries, but the widening of the aorta to its bifurcation does suggest the involvement of the iliac arteries.

What causes an arterial aneurysm? In 95% of cases, the characteristic bulge in the arterial wall results from atherosclerosis. But it can stem instead from trauma, congenital defect, syphilis, cystic medionecrosis, or nonspecific inflammation.

What's common to all aneurysms is damage to the middle or muscular layer of the vessel, the tunica media. With the media's incompetence, the inner (intima) and outer (adventitia) layers of the artery are also helplessly stretched outward. Pressure of the coursing blood as it pounds against the defect can not only enlarge the aneurysm, by exerting relentless pressure on the weakened vessel walls. It can also wear away surrounding structures. In fact, wear and tear on the vessel will ultimately cause its rupture.

Patients with symptoms most commonly complain of pain in the lumbar region radiating into the flank or groin. Such pain stems from pressure on the lumbar nerves. Depending on the atherosclerotic involvement of distal arteries — the iliac and femoral — the patient may complain of symptoms produced by arterial ischemia or occlusion, such as claudication. He may also have abdominal pulsations, GI discomfort, changes in bowel habits, or peripheral edema.

Luckily, 80% of all abdominal aneurysms *are* palpable, so any time you examine an older patient, especially one with vascular disease, keep this in mind. A flat plate of Mr. Rosoff's abdomen revealed a 5-cm aneurysm (a threatening size) with a calcified wall. Since an untreated aneurysm inevitably grows larger, the doctor recommended surgical resection to avoid a potentially fatal rupture.

Rupture?

How do you recognize rupture of an abdominal aneurysm into the peritoneum? Its chief clinical features are pain and signs of blood loss. Many victims feel a sudden and then constant severe pain in the abdomen or pain in the lower back, radiating to the groin. Along with the pain come weakness, sweating, tachycardia, and a drop in blood pressure, either mild or severe enough to signal shock.

If you palpate such a patient's abdomen, you'll no longer feel a discrete aneurysmal wall. Instead, you'll feel a pulsatile heave of the entire retroperitoneum. There won't be time for tests. Once the diagnosis is made, the patient must be rushed to the operating room. No attempt can be made to stabilize him, nor can surgery be postponed. If treated in time, the patient's chances of surviving are about 3 to 2. If not, he will die.

Who's a candidate for surgery? A patient with a lesion less than 6 cm may be treated conservatively (with regular lateral ultrasonography and abdominal X-rays to detect enlargement). Even so, the potential for rupture in a small aneurysm can still be as high as 20%. With a patient who has an aneurysm larger than 6 cm, the risk of rupture is from 40% to 80% within 2 to 5 years of diagnosis. Since aneurysms tend to enlarge, most vascular surgeons recommend resection in all relatively low-risk patients with an aneurysm larger than 6 cm, and in those patients under age 65 with an aneurysm between 4 and 6 cm. A symptomatic aneurysm, of course, warrants immediate

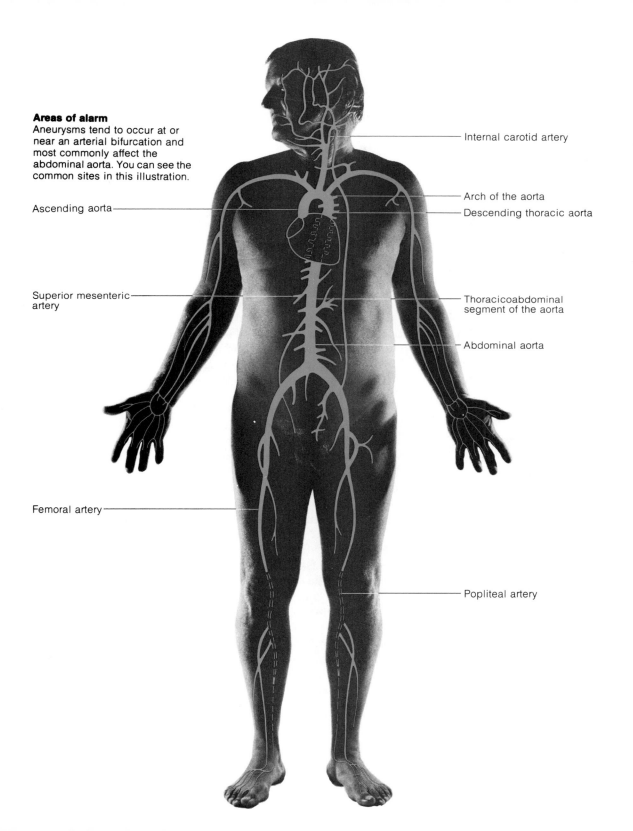

Areas of alarm
Aneurysms tend to occur at or near an arterial bifurcation and most commonly affect the abdominal aorta. You can see the common sites in this illustration.

Internal carotid artery

Ascending aorta

Arch of the aorta

Descending thoracic aorta

Superior mesenteric artery

Thoracicoabdominal segment of the aorta

Abdominal aorta

Femoral artery

Popliteal artery

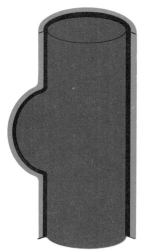

Aneurysms take many forms
Damage to the media layer may
cause the aneurysm to bulge on
only one side of the artery. This
kind is called saccular.

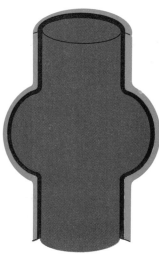

If an aneurysm bulges
out on both sides of the
affected vessel,
it's called a fusiform
aneurysm.

consideration for surgery.

In cases where a rupture is not imminent, however, elective surgery allows time for completion of diagnostic preop tests.

Preop management

The day before elective surgery is filled with tests, consultations, and numerous procedures. Your preop role with aneurysm patients can be strong: obtaining baseline data (vital signs, the character of peripheral pulses, breath sounds, and so on), taking a history, explaining the various procedures involved, and offering the patient and his family support to reduce their anxiety.

Before Mr. Rosoff was taken to the O.R. we took a complete set of vital signs and inserted an I.V. and a Foley catheter. We weighed him on the ICU bed scale to obtain a baseline weight: Any change would guide fluid management (a crucial consideration before, during, and after surgery). An arterial line and a central venous pressure (CVP) line were inserted. If the patient has heart disease, a pulmonary artery catheter allows continuous monitoring of PAP and PWP. Remember that CVP monitoring measures right heart pressure and may not accurately reflect pressure on the left side of the heart. Along with other preop medications, we gave him cephalothin (Keflin), a broad-spectrum antibiotic, which would be continued for 48 hours postoperatively to prevent infection.

Postop management complex

In the O.R., the surgeon resected the aneurysm and inserted a Dacron bifurcation graft. It extended from below the renal arteries to the femoral arteries. Mr. Rosoff was transferred to the ICU with an endotracheal tube, a Salem sump nasogastric tube, a CVP line, an arterial line, and a Foley catheter all in place. We hung an I.V., with 5% dextrose in ½ normal saline with 20 mEq potassium. Then we placed him on a MA-1 volume-controlled ventilator, and connected him to the cardiac monitor. We sent blood for a complete blood count, electrolytes, BUN, creatinine, and ABGs. Then we started an ICU flow sheet to monitor and record his vital signs and his hemodynamic, respiratory, and neurologic status, as well as his fluid intake and output.

Our next job: to take a complete set of Mr. Rosoff's vital signs. His rectal temperature on admission to the ICU was

99.4° F. (37.4° C.); heart rate, 94; blood pressure, 120/60; and CVP, 10 cm H$_2$O. (To prevent the declamping hypotension phenomenon, the patient's vascular volume is kept to the maximum point on his Starling curve during surgery.) We checked his popliteal, pedal, and posterior tibial pulses every hour at first, recording them on the flow sheet. We also noted the temperature, color, and movement of his legs. (A decreased or absent pulse along with cool, mottled extremities would have indicated embolization — or even occlusion of the graft). Also, to watch for internal bleeding, we measured and recorded his abdominal girth every 2 hours.

Fortunately, renal failure — once a common complication of abdominal aneurysm resection — is now rare. But you need to know the urine output just to ensure adequate renal perfusion. If it's less than 30 ml per hour for 2 consecutive hours, notify the doctor. Check the urine for specific gravity at least every 3 or 4 hours. If the patient becomes hypovolemic, his kidneys will try to conserve salt and water by producing only small amounts of concentrated urine. Its specific gravity will be more than 1.030. Mr. Rosoff's urine reached a specific gravity of 1.025, high normal.

We checked for evidence of emboli in his legs due to necrotic debris and monitored the EKG carefully, watching for changes consistent with ischemia. In older patients with atherosclerosis, like Mr. Rosoff, the potential for CVA means that you must check neurologic vital signs not only in the initial assessment but also every 2 to 3 hours thereafter. About an hour after admission to the ICU, Mr. Rosoff was awake, alert, and oriented. He showed an equal reaction to light in his pupils, had a good grip in either hand, and remained stable.

Respiratory care crucial

Because many such patients have a history of pulmonary disease, possibly because of their age, you must assess their respiratory status frequently. You must be proficient in auscultating breath sounds and identifying any adventitious sounds such as rales, which may denote fluid in the alveoli.

Many aneurysm patients develop adult respiratory distress syndrome from 24 to 48 hours postop. This seems to result from an inflammatory response to the massive resection, which builds a large amount of fluid in the retroperitoneal space. A day or two postop, this fluid may start leaking into the

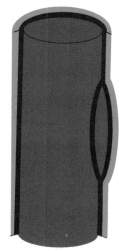

Blood splitting vessel layers, a dissecting aneurysm, commonly affects the thoracic aorta. It's associated with connective tissue disorders or trauma.

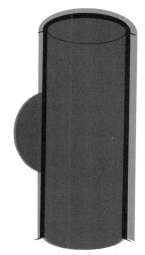

When all vessel layers rupture, as in trauma, this is called a false aneurysm. (A true aneurysm has one layer intact.) Escaping blood forms a pulsating hematoma.

interstitial spaces of the lung. But usually this complication can be prevented with a diuretic, such as furosemide (Lasix).

We were careful to turn Mr. Rosoff every 2 hours, suction his endotracheal tube as needed, and take blood for gas determinations at regular intervals. Besides an EKG, we took a chest X-ray as soon as possible after surgery and repeated it daily while he was in the ICU. Mr. Rosoff assisted the respirator minimally. We suctioned him for moderate amounts of white sputum. Breath sounds were present bilaterally, and we heard a few bibasilar rales. We were eager to avoid respiratory alkalosis from overuse of the ventilator. Such alkalosis would increase the affinity of oxygen for the hemoglobin molecule and so impede its use by the tissues. Mr. Rosoff's blood gases were normal: PO_2, 126; PCO_2, 38; pH, 7.45. We adjusted the FIO_2 on the ventilator accordingly.

Most aneurysm repair patients remain intubated for 24 hours after surgery. They can be extubated and started on oxygen by mask when they can generate an adequate tidal volume, vital capacity, peak inspiratory force... and when their ABGs are normal while being weaned from the ventilator. Then they need chest physiotherapy, nasotracheal suction, and early mobilization. Help them by giving analgesics beforehand and by splinting the incision with pillows during coughing exercises.

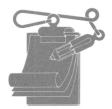

Remember these important points about aneurysms:
1. Observe your patient for signs of aortic aneurysm rupture: for example, pain in the abdomen or lower back radiating to the groin, weakness, sweating, tachycardia, and a drop in blood pressure.
2. When examining an elderly patient, especially one with vascular disease, be sure to palpate for an abdominal aneurysm. Although your patient may be asymptomatic, most abdominal aneurysms are palpable.
3. Be aware that regular lateral ultrasonography and abdominal X-rays help monitor aneurysm size.
4. When indicated, prepare your patient for an aneurysm resection by obtaining baseline data, taking a history, explaining the procedures involved, and offering support and reassurance.
5. Following surgery, take vital signs at least hourly, check urine output hourly, watch for EKG changes, and assess respiratory status. Report any abnormalities immediately.

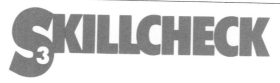

SKILLCHECK

1. A 67-year-old retired lawyer, Mike Loger, is a patient on your unit. He tells you that he has pain in both legs after walking 6 to 8 blocks. His pain goes away within a few minutes after he rests. Would you suspect: arterial insufficiency, venous insufficiency, osteoarthritis, or neuropathy?

2. How can you confirm Mr. Loger's diagnosis and assess his degree of insufficiency?

3. Marie Wade has been a waitress for the past 23 years. She has just been admitted to your unit for an evaluation of her varicose veins. Do you think her varicosities are superficial or deep? How can you make the distinction?

4. Which of the following symptoms indicates venous insufficiency: leg cramps at night; leg pain (claudication) after walking 6 to 8 blocks that is relieved by resting for a brief period of time; nodules or ropelike formation in the legs; or painful swelling in the calves?

5. What relieves venous symptoms? Smoking, resting, walking, or dangling the legs?

6. What causes leg ulcers? Ischemia secondary to arterial insufficiency; stasis secondary to venous insufficiency; or both?

7. How are abdominal aneurysms detectable? By auscultation, by palpation, by inspection, or by percussion?

8. Abdominal aneurysms are most likely to occur in persons...over 60; 40 to 60; under 40?

9. What causes arterial aneurysms?

10. True or false: When all vessel layers rupture, this is called a fusiform aneurysm.

(Answers on page 172)

SKILLCHECK ANSWERS

ANSWERS TO SKILLCHECK 1 (page 41)

Situation 1
Sally has a water-hammer, or Corrigan's, pulse. It probably indicates patent ductus arteriosus (PDA), although it's also found with aortic regurgitation.

Situation 2
In children the diastolic blood pressure is the point at which the pulse sounds become muffled. Some institutions record all three sounds (e.g., 108/70/50).

Situation 3
A low-pitched sound immediately following S_2 and heard best at the apex is an S_3. If it's caused by ventricular abnormality, it's called a ventricular gallop; but it's frequently heard in children and young adults with normal cardiac function. S_3 is caused by the vibrations in the ventricles rapidly filling with blood. Record this finding in your notes. You need not notify the doctor unless there are other signs of cardiac disease.

Situation 4
This pattern is termed sinus arrhythmia. During inspiration, a greater volume of blood is drawn into the pulmonary vessels, decreasing the flow of pulmonary blood into the left atrium and left ventricle. The heart rate automatically increases to make up for the lower cardiac output. During expiration, when the cardiac output is higher, the heart rate slows. Sinus arrhythmia is normal in both children and adults.

Situation 5
An S_3 on auscultation.

Situation 6
Aortic stenosis.

Situation 7
Polycythemia.

Situation 8
The mechanism is different in the two kinds of cardiac anomalies. In acyanotic defects (VSD, ASD, PDA, and coarctation of the aorta), the left-to-right shunt produces pulmonary system overload and interstitial edema. The edema, a good culture medium for bacteria, predisposes the child to frequent respiratory in-fections. In cyanotic defects (tetralogy of Fallot, transposition of the great vessels), some or all of the circulating blood bypasses the lung's cleansing filtration. This predisposes to respiratory complications.

Situation 9
Low cardiac output.

Situation 10
Start oxygen. The PVCs may be caused by myocardial ischemia. Document the arrhythmia with EKG strips and take a 12-lead EKG to make sure that they're ventricular ectopics. Once you've established this diagnosis, give antiarrhythmic medication and notify the doctor immediately. See that a serum potassium level is drawn — Paul may have hypokalemia. The PVCs may also be related to the surgical procedure.

ANSWERS TO SKILLCHECK 2 (page 151)

Situation 1
Hypertension makes the heart work harder as a result of constricted peripheral circulation. It also increases atherogenic tendencies.

Situation 2
Myocardial nerve endings transmit pain to the upper thoracic posterior roots.

Situation 3
All of these patients may get a pulmonary embolus, but the last patient is most at risk because of his long immobilization. An immobile patient's blood flow is decreased 50% with pooling in dependent body areas from generalized vasodilation. Decreased blood flow and pooling are major causes of thrombus formation.

Situation 4
Several complications could explain Martha's symptoms: myocardial infarction, pericarditis, pneumonia, bronchitis, an episode of supraventricular tachycardia, or pulmonary embolus. Any one of these is possible. But Martha's immobilization for over 3 weeks makes pulmonary embolus or pneumonia the most likely. A lung scan would differentiate between them.

Obtain a blood sample for arterial blood gases. Then elevate the head of the bed to 45° and administer oxygen by mask or nasal cannula. Notify her doctor.

While awaiting orders, start an I.V. (in case shock develops and for the possible administration of anticoagulant medication and digitalis) and do an EKG. Reassure the patient and do not leave her alone.

Situation 5
John's optic fundi show an advanced stage of malignant hypertension. The prognosis is grave, and his condition requires vigorous medical management.

Situation 6
CPK-MB.

Situation 7
S-T depression.

Situation 8
Inderal reduces myocardial oxygen consumption by decreasing heart rate and contractility.

Situation 9
Nausea and vomiting are common vagal responses to AMI pain and may also be side effects of morphine. Usually these symptoms end spontaneously. Remember, however, that persistent vomiting can cause potassium depletion (lost in the gastric contents). Hypokalemia can cause arrhythmias. Since the AMI patient is already at risk for life-threatening arrhythmias, make sure serum potassium levels are within normal limits if a patient has been vomiting. He may need a potassium supplement.

Situation 10
You hear three heart sounds in the following order: S_4, S_1, S_2. S_4 (atrial gallop) occurs at the end of ventricular diastole when the atria contract and send a bolus of blood into an already blood-filled ventricle. If the left ventricle is stiff (noncompliant) because of the infarction, the vibrations from the blood entering the ventricle are transmitted to the chest wall as a low-pitched sound. Almost all AMI patients have S_4 during the first couple of days. However, chart it in your notes.

Situation 11
All three of the cardiac enzymes (SGOT, LDH, and CPK) occur in skeletal muscle as well as in the myocardium. Give all pain medication intravenously. Intramuscular injections cause irregular absorption and may raise enzyme levels.

Situation 12
John's decreased level of consciousness and vital signs all point to cardiac tamponade. Suspect rupture of the heart (a fatal complication of AMI). This is an *extreme emergency*. Even with quick intervention, the patient's prognosis is very poor.

ANSWERS TO SKILLCHECK 3 (page 169)

Situation 1
Most likely, Mr. Loger has arterial insufficiency. In venous insufficiency, leg pain usually gets better with walking, not worse; in osteoarthritis or neuropathy, the pain usually persists, even after rest. Mr. Loger has the classic symptoms of arterial insufficiency: His leg pain comes on exertion and goes away within a few minutes upon resting.

Situation 2
Doppler ultrasonography shows diminished circulation and supports a diagnosis of arterial insufficiency.

Situation 3
Having had a job that required prolonged standing and walking for a number of years supports a diagnosis of primary, or superficial, varicosities. Phlebography is used to distinguish between primary and secondary (deep thrombophlebitis) varicosities.

Situation 4
Leg cramps at night, nodules or ropelike formations in the legs, and swollen calves.

Situation 5
Walking relieves venous symptoms.

Situation 6
Both ischemic and venous stasis are causes of leg ulcers.

Situation 7
Palpation: 80% of abdominal aneurysms are palpable.

Situation 8
Abdominal aneurysms usually occur in persons over age 60.

Situation 9
In 95% of cases, arterial aneurysms result from atherosclerosis. Other causes: trauma, congenital defect, syphilis, cystic medionecrosis, or inflammation.

Situation 10
False. A fusiform aneurysm is one that bulges out on both sides of an affected vessel. When all vessel layers rupture, this is called a false aneurysm.

Appendices

CARDIAC REHABILITATION PLAN
FOR GRADUATED ACTIVITY AND EXERCISE

IN HOSPITAL	EXERCISE	ACTIVITY
Day 2	Passive range of motion (ROM) to all extremities in bed; active plantar extension and dorsiflexion	Bedside commode; feed self; groom self
Days 3 and 4	Active ROM (up to 10X)	Bathe self under supervision.
Days 5 to 7	Minimal resistance to active ROM 10X each	Walk back and forth in room twice q.i.d.
Days 8 and 9	Moderate resistance to active ROM 10X each	Stand at sink to shave; walk to bathroom under observation p.r.n.
Day 10	Add: Exercise: Three arm and shoulder motions, five lateral bends and knee raises, and five side leg raises	Take a shower; walk in hall b.i.d.
Days 11 and 12	Add: Sitting on flat bed, touch toes, and twist trunk twice	Sit up most of day; walk length of hall b.i.d.
Days 13 and 14	Add: Three standing half knee bends	Walk at will, including up and down one flight of stairs.

The above regimen is done under the direct supervision of the cardiac rehabilitation team. The activities should terminate whenever the pulse rate exceeds 115 BPM, ectopic beats occur, or the patient experiences chest pain.

SOME HEART-SAVING ADVICE FOR PATIENTS AFTER DISCHARGE

Eat 4 small meals a day; eat them slowly.

Avoid situations, people, and conditions that make you tense, upset, or angry.

Plan your activities to allow your heart to rest:
—Plan and spread out your work to avoid overload and allow rest between chores.
—If you get tired, no matter what you are doing, stop and rest for 15 to 20 minutes. Don't push yourself to finish mowing the grass, or watch the last 30 minutes of that television show.
—Try not to hurry.
—Plan a 30-minute rest period twice a day.
—Get 6 to 8 hours sleep each night.
—Avoid working with arms above shoulder level. Don't wash windows or hang clothes on the line.

During the first weeks at home continue to be as active as you were on the last day in the hospital. You can do the following things: Get up and get dressed every day.

Walk daily, as much as you were walking in the hospital. You may walk outside when the weather is nice but walk on level ground. Avoid steps and hills. Avoid walking against the wind because your heart works harder and beats faster then. In the winter, walk during the warmest part of the day; in the summer, walk in the morning or evening when it is cool. Walk after a rest period, or when you are not tired. If you have chest discomfort or shortness of breath, stop and sit down on the steps or curb, take nitroglycerin if you have some, and wait until you feel OK again. Tell your doctor about this pain when you see him.

Climb stairs only once a day. You may need to take only a few steps at a time and stop and rest. Avoid doing anything which tenses your body, such as:
• straining when having a bowel movement (ask your doctor about a laxative)
• lifting anything heavy — children, groceries, or suitcases
• pushing or pulling anything heavy
• trying to open a stuck window or unscrew a stuck jar lid.

During later weeks home
Ask your doctor when you may:
• drive the car
• return to work
• go fishing
• go to the movies
• go to a ball game
• roll up your hair.
You may cut the lawn with a self-propelled mower or riding mower. Do this activity with care and in cool weather.

When your doctor says you may work, try to arrange to go back part time at first and then slowly increase your working time.

You may have other questions about your activities, diet, medication, or illness. If you do, feel free to ask your doctor.

General advice
If you develop pain, numbness, or shortness of breath, stop what you are doing, take your nitroglycerin, and rest for several minutes. When the discomfort disappears, continue what you were doing at a slower rate.

Follow your fat-controlled diet. It is an important part of the doctor's plan to help reduce your blood cholesterol.

Continue the physical therapy exercises started in the hospital until you return to normal activity. Do these exercises twice daily.

After a meal, your heart is already working to digest your food. Therefore, rest for an hour after eating before doing any heavy exercise.

Stop smoking. Smoking cigarettes increases your chance of having another heart attack.

If your doctor says you may have liquor, drink in moderation.

Check with your doctor before you take a long trip. As you travel, stop every two hours and walk around to prevent clots from forming in your lower legs. Also, check with your doctor before going to the mountains or to a hot, humid place. Airplane trips are usually permitted one month after your discharge.

As with other activities you should not have sex if:
• you are tired — take a 30-minute nap first
• you have just eaten a heavy meal
• you have been drinking
• you are angry with your mate
• the temperature of the room is uncomfortably warm or cool.
If you begin to have chest discomfort, STOP. The next time, try taking nitroglycerin beforehand. Remember, it's normal for your heart to beat faster and your breathing to speed up during sexual activity. Your heart beat and breathing should slow down and return to normal shortly afterward.

Notify your doctor immediately whenever you have:
• heavy pressure or squeezing pain in the chest which may spread to the shoulder, arm, neck, or jaw and is not relieved in 15 minutes by resting and/or nitroglycerin
• increased shortness of breath
• unusual tiredness
• swelling of feet and ankles
• fainting
• very slow or rapid heart rate.

SOME CARDIOVASCULAR DRUGS

DRUG	USE, ROUTE, AND DOSAGE	SIDE EFFECTS	NURSING TIPS
atropine sulfate	Anticholinergic (for bradycardia) — I.V. bolus 0.5 mg; may repeat	Therapeutic dosages: dry mouth, cycloplegia, and mydriasis. Large dosages: hyperpyrexia, urinary retention, confusion, and hallucinations	• When protocol allows, give to patients with bradycardia (rate < 50 BPM) who have hypotension, syncope, dyspnea, or ventricular arrhythmias.
clonidine hydrochloride Catapres ◊	Antihypertensive — P.O.: initial dose 0.1 mg b.i.d.; increase by 0.1 to 0.2 mg/day until desired response obtained; usual maintenance dose is 0.2 to 0.8 mg daily in divided doses	Dry mouth, drowsiness, sedation, constipation, dizziness, headache, fatigue	• Don't discontinue abruptly. • Warn patient about sedative effect. • Patient should not drink alcohol or take sedatives with this drug.
calcium chloride	Cardiac stimulant — I.V. bolus, intracardiac 1 g (10 ml of a 10% solution); may repeat	Cardiac arrhythmia (in digitalized patients), venous irritation, vasodilation, hypotension, bradycardia, syncope, and cardiac arrest	• Very irritating; take extreme care to avoid extravasation when giving I.V. • Avoid using in digitalized patients; may cause fatal arrhythmia.
dopamine hydrochloride Intropin ◊	Adrenergic, inotropic agent — I.V. infusion 5 mcg/kg/min up to 50 mcg/kg/min	Ectopic beats, tachycardia, angina, palpitation, vasoconstriction, hypotension, dyspnea, nausea and vomiting, and headache	• Do not add to alkaline solutions; for example, sodium bicarbonate. • Monitor EKG for ventricular arrhythmias. • Check urine output q 30 min. • Rate of infusion is adjusted according to cardiac output, peripheral perfusion, urine output, and pulmonary and arterial pressures; monitor all these parameters closely. • Must be diluted to 250- to 500-ml volume before using.
disopyramide (base or phosphate) Norpace ◊ Rythmodan ◊ ◊	Antiarrhythmic — P.O.: loading dose 300 mg, then 100 to 150 mg q6h	Dry mouth, eyes, nose, throat; urinary hesitancy or retention; urinary frequency or urgency; GI distress; constipation; blurred vision; weight gain (edema); headache; generalized fatigue and weakness; dizziness; rash; nervousness; hypotension; shortness of breath; chest pain; and syncope	• Don't give to patients in cardiogenic shock, second- or third-degree AV block. • Give cautiously to patients with renal or liver disease. • If hypotension or heart failure occurs, notify the doctor immediately.

Guide to this chart:
◊   Also available in Canada.
◊ ◊ Available in Canada only.

(continued on next page)

SOME CARDIOVASCULAR DRUGS *(continued)*

DRUG	USE, ROUTE, AND DOSAGE	SIDE EFFECTS	NURSING TIPS
epinephrine hydrochloride Adrenalin	Adrenergic, cardiac stimulant — I.V. bolus, intracardiac 0.5 to 1 mg (5 to 10 ml of 1:10,000 sol); may repeat	Fear, anxiety, headache, tremor, dizziness, disorientation, nausea and vomiting, sweating, pallor, respiratory difficulty and apnea, palpitations, tachycardia, angina, ventricular arrhythmias	• Watch for pulmonary edema due to peripheral vasoconstriction. • Stop if headache, chest pain, nausea, or hypotension occur. • I.V. injection of 1:1,000 solution leads to hypertension, subarachnoid hemorrhage, and hemiplegia.
digoxin Lanoxin ◇	Congestive heart failure, atrial fibrillation and flutter, paroxysmal atrial tachycardia — Loading dose: 0.5 to 1 mg I.V. or P.O. in divided doses over 24 hours; maintenance 0.125 to 0.5 mg I.V. or P.O. daily (average 0.25 mg; however, less in elderly patients and those with renal insufficiency); larger doses often needed for treatment of arrhythmias, depending on patient response	Fatigue, generalized muscle weakness, agitation, hallucinations, headache, malaise, dizziness, vertigo, stupor, paresthesias, increased severity of congestive heart failure, arrhythmias, hypotension, yellow-green halos around visual images, blurred vision, light flashes, photophobia, diplopia, anorexia, nausea, vomiting, and diarrhea	• Obtain baseline data before giving first dose. • Monitor serum potassium carefully. • Take apical-radial pulse for a full minute. Record and report to doctor any significant changes. • Excessive slowing of pulse rate (60/min or less) may be sign of digoxin toxicity. • Drug is contraindicated in presence of any digitalis-induced toxicity, ventricular fibrillation, or ventricular tachycardia, unless caused by congestive heart failure. • Use cautiously in patients with acute myocardial infarction; incomplete AV block; chronic constrictive pericarditis; idiopathic, hypertropic subaortic stenosis; renal insufficiency; severe pulmonary disease; hypothyroidism; and in the elderly.
hydralazine hydrochloride Apresoline ◇ Rolazine	Afterload reducer, antihypertensive — P.O.: Initial dose 10 mg q.i.d. for 4 days, then 25 mg q.i.d. for 3 days, then 50 mg q.i.d. thereafter. Maintenance: lowest effective dose I.V., I.M.: 20 to 40 mg repeated as necessary	Headache, palpitations, GI disturbance, tachycardia, angina, flushing, peripheral neuritis, edema, anxiety, lupus-like syndrome	• Watch for signs of myocardial ischemia: angina, and EKG changes. • Use cautiously in patients with suspected coronary artery disease.
isoproterenol hydrochloride Isuprel ◇	Beta-adrenergic, cardiac stimulant — I.V. bolus, intracardiac 0.02 mg; I.V. infusion	Arrhythmias, palpitations, tachycardia, headache, flushing, dizziness, sweating, and tremors	• Slow or stop infusion if heart rate exceeds 110/min. • Discontinue if ventricular arrhythmia occurs.

SOME CARDIOVASCULAR DRUGS *(continued)*

DRUG	USE, ROUTE, AND DOSAGE	SIDE EFFECTS	NURSING TIPS
isoproterenol hydrochloride *(continued)*	of 1 mg/500 ml D_5W titrated to heart rate and blood pressure		• Have defibrillator at bedside. • Measure urine output and B.P. every 15 min. • Do not use concurrently with epinephrine; may cause serious arrhythmias.
lidocaine hydrochloride Xylocaine ◊	Ventricular antiarrhythmic — I.V. bolus 100 mg followed by I.V. infusion 1 to 2 g/500 ml D_5W at 1 to 4 mg/min; may repeat bolus q 3 to 5 min. Don't exceed 300 mg total bolus during 1 hr.	Hypotension, cardiovascular collapse, bradycardia, convulsions, respiratory depression, visual disturbances, and slurred speech. Severe reactions may be preceeded by somnolence and paresthesia	• Give cautiously to patients with Stokes-Adams syndrome, liver disease, or CHF; may cause toxicity. • If CNS side effects occur, stop the infusion immediately, give O_2, and call the doctor.
metaraminol bitartrate Aramine	Alpha- and beta-adrenergic, vasopressor — I.V. 15 to 100 mg/500 ml D_5/NSS. Adjust rate to maintain B.P.	Anxiety, tremor, faintness, headache, dizziness, precordial pain, respiratory difficulty, flushing, pallor, sweating, and nausea	• Monitor vital signs q 30 min. • MAO inhibitors potentiate its pressor effect. • Guanethidine-metaraminol interaction may cause hypertensive crisis.
methyldopa Aldomet ◊	Antihypertensive — P.O.: Initial dose 250 mg b.i.d. or t.i.d. for 2 days, then increase or decrease dose every 2 days until desired effect obtained. Maintenance: 500 mg to 3 g daily in 2 to 4 doses. I.V. infusion: 250 to 500 mg (maximum dose 1 g) in 100 ml D_5W over 30 to 60 min q6h (dose titrated according to B.P.)	Sedation, headache, and weakness (all transient); orthostatic hypotension; edema; GI distress; liver function test abnormalities; positive Coombs' test; drug fever; rash; impotence; dry mouth; and nasal stuffiness	• Use cautiously in patients with liver disease. • Warn patients about sedative effect. • Baseline blood count recommended at start and periodically during therapy.
nitroprusside sodium Nipride ◊	Vasodilator, antihypertensive — I.V. 0.5 to 10 mcg/kg/min continuous I.V. infusion. Use only D_5W for dilution; to make solution containing 100 mcg/ml, dilute 50 mg nitroprusside in 500 ml D_5W	GI disturbance, increased perspiration, headache, restlessness, apprehension, muscle twitching, retrosternal discomfort, palpitations, dizziness, hypotension, and irritation at infusion site	• Protect container from light — wrap in foil. • Prepare fresh infusion q4h. • Use infusion pump. • Avoid extravasation. • Monitor vital signs q 5 min while the infusion is being started then q 15 min. • Discard solution after 24 hr.

(continued on next page)

SOME CARDIOVASCULAR DRUGS *(continued)*

DRUG	USE, ROUTE, AND DOSAGE	SIDE EFFECTS	NURSING TIPS
norepinephrine injection (formerly levarterenol bitartrate) Levophed ◊	Alpha- and beta-adrenergic, vasopressor — I.V. infusion 8 to 16 mg (2 to 4 amps) in 500 ml D$_5$W titrated to blood pressure	Intense sweating, vomiting, severe hypertension, headache, weakness, dizziness, tremor, pallor, respiratory difficulty, precordial pain, cardiac arrhythmias, and tissue necrosis and sloughing from extravasation of injection	• Check infusion site frequently to avoid extravasation. Should extravasation occur, stop infusion and flush the area immediately with 15 ml of saline solution and 10 ml of phentolamine to avoid sloughing of tissue. • Guanethidine and methyldopa increase norepinephrine's effect.
prazosin hydrochloride Minipress ◊	Vasodilator, antihypertensive — P.O.: Initial dose 1 mg t.i.d. Maintenance: 3 to 20 mg daily in divided doses (a few patients may require up to 40 mg daily)	Severe syncope may occur if initial dose greater than 1 mg; headache, drowsiness, weakness, palpitations, GI disturbance, edema, dry mouth, and dizziness	• Observe closely for syncopal episodes after initial dose and each dosage increase. Such episodes usually occur within 60 to 90 min after dose. • Administer intial dose at bedtime to minimize effect of syncope.
procainamide hydrochloride Pronestyl ◊	Ventricular antiarrhythmic — P.O.: 250 to 500 mg q3 to 4h I.M.: 0.5 to 1 g q6h until patient can take drug P.O. I.V.: 100 mg q5 min (at rate of 20 to 50 mg/min) up to maximum loading dose of 1g or until arrhythmia suppressed. Drip of 2 to 6 mg/min may be used after loading dose.	Hypotension and serious disturbances of cardiac rhythm due to Q-T prolongation with I.M. or I.V. routes: GI disturbances, urticaria, pruritus, fever, chills, weakness, depression, psychosis, lupus-like syndrome and positive ANA test (during prolonged therapy), and agranulocytosis	• Watch for cardiac arrhythmias, atrial fibrillation, and ventricular tachycardia after I.V. administration. • Tell patient to report any sore throat or sores in mouth, unexplained fever, or upper respiratory tract infection. • Use I.V. route only for emergencies.
propranolol hydrochloride Inderal ◊ Inderal LA ◊	Antihypertensive, antianginal, antiarrhythmic — P.O.: Hypertension, 80 to 640 mg daily in divided doses; or sustained-release capsule once daily. Angina and arrhythmias, 10 to 40 mg q.i.d. I.V: 1 to 3 mg	Bradycardia, CHF, intensification of AV block, hypotension, light-headedness, visual disturbances, GI distress, bronchospasm; exacerbation of angina and MI may follow abrupt withdrawal of drug; and mental disturbances ranging from disorientation to catatonia	• Do not discontinue abruptly. • Note small I.V. dose compared to P.O. dose. • Use I.V. route only for life-threatening arrhythmias. • Drug may mask signs of hypoglycemia in diabetic patients.
quinidine bisulfate Biquin Durules ◊ ◊ **quinidine gluconate** Duraquin, Quinaglute Dura-Tabs ◊ , Quinate ◊ ◊	Atrial and ventricular antiarrhythmic — P.O.: 200 to 400 mg q4 to 6h I.M.: Initial dose 300 to 400 mg, then 200 mg q2h times four (for	Tinnitus, headache, disturbed vision, cardiac asystole, ventricular arrhythmias, widening of QRS complex, paradoxical tachycardia, GI disturbance, vertigo, excitement, confusion, cutaneous flushing with intense	• Give test dose (200 mg) to determine idiosyncrasy; observe patient closely; take vital signs frequently. • Give cautiously to patients in incomplete AV block (may cause complete AV

SOME CARDIOVASCULAR DRUGS *(continued)*

DRUG	USE, ROUTE, AND DOSAGE	SIDE EFFECTS	NURSING TIPS
quinidine *(continued)* **quinidine polyga-lacturonate** Cardioquin ◊ **quinidine sulfate** CinQuin, Quine, Quinidex Extentabs, Quinora, SK-Quinidine Sulfate	acute tachycardia)	pruritus, hypersensitivity reaction, and fever	block). • Widening of QRS complex by 50% is sign of quinidine cardiotoxicity. Stop drug immediately.
reserpine Serpasil ◊ Reserpanca ◊ ◊	Antihypertensive — P.O.: Initial dose 0.5 mg daily for 1 to 2 weeks. Maintenance 0.1 to 0.5 mg daily. I.M.: Initial dose 0.5 to 1 mg, then 2 to 4 mg q3h until desired response	Depression, GI disturbances including hypersecretion, angina-like symptoms, arrhythmias, drowsiness, nervousness, anxiety, nightmares, dull sensorium, deafness, nasal congestion, pruritus, rash, dry mouth, dizziness, headache, impotence, dysuria, myalgias, and edema	• Use cautiously in patients with renal disease (lowered B.P. may further compromise renal function). • Avoid in patients with history of mental depression. • Watch closely for signs of developing despondency. • Contraindicated in patients with ulcer disease or ulcerative colitis.
sodium bicarbonate	To prevent acidosis — I.V. bolus 1 mEq/kg; repeat in 10 min, if necessary. Further doses based on blood gas analysis. If ABGs unavailable, use 0.5 mEq/kg every 10 min during resuscitation	Metabolic alkalosis	• Incompatible with calcium solutions. • A 4.2% solution, slow administration, is preferred for children under age 2. • Watch for signs of alkalosis: nausea, vomiting, diarrhea, slow and shallow respirations, confusion, irritability, and twitching.
verapamil	Calcium channel blocker, antiarrhythmic — I.V. push 0.075 to 0.15 mg/kg (5 to 10 mg) over 60 seconds with EKG and blood pressure monitoring. Repeat dose in 30 minutes if no response. Follow bolus injection with maintenance infusion of 0.005 mg/kg/min.	Dizziness, headache, transient hypotension, heart failure, bradycardia, AV block, ventricular systole, and constipation	• Give cautiously to patients with myocardial infarction followed by coronary occlusion, sick sinus syndrome, impaired AV conduction, and heart failure with atrial tachyarrhythmia. • Note that patients with severely compromised cardiac function or those receiving beta blockers should receive lower doses. • Contraindicated in patients with advanced heart failure, AV block, cardiogenic shock, sinus node disease, and severe hypotension. • Drug should not be given within 30 minutes if patient received I.V. beta blocker; both cause myocardial depression.

Glossary

acidosis — a condition in which excessive hydrogen ions (pH) are present in body fluids due to loss of base or retention of noncarbonic acids.

akinesis — temporary paralysis or failure of part of the cardiac muscle to contract during systole.

alkalosis — opposite of acidosis; occurs with decreased hydrogen ion (pH) concentration in body fluids due to loss of acid or retention of base.

amyloid — a waxy, translucent, insoluble glycoprotein; occurs in many conditions and leaves tissues waxy and nonfunctional.

anasarca — generalized massive edema.

aneurysm — a sac formed by the bulging wall of an artery or vein.

angina pectoris — chest pain due to insufficient delivery of oxygen to the myocardium. Status anginosus — angina occuring at rest and resistant to treatment.

angiogram — visualization of a blood vessel after injection of a contrast medium.

angiotensin — a vasoconstrictor found in blood.

anoxia — oxygen deficiency in body tissue due to reduced blood flow or other causes, resulting in tissue injury or death.

anticholinergic — an effect that blocks impulse transmission across the parasympathetic ganglia; a substance that blocks the effects of acetylcholine.

arrhythmia — any disturbance in rate, rhythm, or conduction of the heart.

arteriography — visualization of an artery (arteries) after injection of a radiopaque material into the bloodstream.

arteriosclerosis — a group of diseases that result in thickening and loss of elasticity of arterial walls.

ascites — abnormal accumulation of fluid in the abdominal cavity.

asynchronism — disturbance of the time factor in the cardiac contraction sequence.

atelectasis — collapse of all or part of a lung.

atherosclerosis — narrowing of the lumen of arterial walls via the accumulation of fatty plaques.

atrioventricular (AV) node — a group of specialized cardiac muscle fibers located in the floor of the right atrium that carries electrical impulses from the atria to the bundle of His.

autoimmune — immunologic action against the body's own tissue.

bigeminal rhythm — beats that occur in pairs — one normal, one premature (supraventricular or ventricular).

bradycardia — abnormal slowness of heart rate; usually fewer than 60 beats/minute.

Buerger's disease — a chronic recurring inflammatory disease affecting the arteries and veins, especially in the legs. Also know as thromboangiitis obliterans.

bundle of His — group of specialized muscle fibers in the interventricular septum of the heart; conveys electrical impulses from the AV node to the Purkinje's fibers to stimulate ventricular contraction.

cardiac catheterization — a diagnostic test in which a catheter is introduced into a blood vessel and maneuvered into the heart. The purpose of this procedure is to obtain blood samples from the heart, detect abnormalities, and determine intracardiac pressure.

cardiac cycle — one heartbeat; time required for heart to complete filling (diastole) and emptying (systole) — usually 8/10 of a second.

cardiac output — force and volume of blood pumped out of the heart per minute.

cardiomegaly — enlarged heart muscle. Chambers generally remain normal size with excess tissue accumulation.

cardiomyopathy — general term meaning disease of the heart muscle, usually of unknown etiology.

cardioversion — restoration of rapid, abnormal rates and/or rhythms to normal sinus rhythm by drug or electrical countershock.

carotid sinus —a dilated portion of the common carotid artery, just above the bifurcation of the two main branches, containing a rich supply of nerve endings from the sinus branch of the vagus nerve.

central venous pressure (CVP) — the pressure exerted by the blood in the venae cavae and right atrium.

Chagas' disease — a form of trypanosomiasis prevalent in Central and South America. Also called Chagas-Cruz disease, it is transmitted by the reduviid bug.

Cheyne-Stokes respiration — abnormal pattern characterized by slow, shallow breathing that increases in depth and rapidity until it reaches an apex from which it decreases gradually and ceases altogether for a short period; cycle then resumes.

claudication — pain in legs during walking due to inadequate blood supply or venous drainage. Pain subsides with rest.

clubbing — occurs with congenital heart disease and chronic pulmonary disease when the ends of the fingers or toes become swollen and soft and take on a rounded appearance.

coarctation — narrowing or constriction of a vessel; of aorta: causes increased cardiac activity, hypertension in the arms, and hypotension in the legs.

collateral — alternate vascular route formed when original becomes obstructed or reduced.

colloid — a substance which, when in solution, remains suspended, neither dissolving nor settling.

coronary angiography — X-ray examination of the coronary arteries after a radiopaque dye has been injected into them.

coronary arteries — two arteries arising from the aorta that supply the heart with blood.

coronary occlusion — an obstruction or narrowing of one of the coronary arteries, which inhibits the flow of blood to some part of the heart muscle.

cor pulmonale — a serious condition in which increased pressure within the pulmonary artery results in right ventricular heart failure.

creatine phosphokinase (CPK) — an enzyme found in the skeletal muscles, heart, and brain that is released by inflammatory processes.

creatinine — a normal, alkaline, nonprotein end product of metabolism present in the blood and urine.

crystalloid — a substance capable of forming crystals and of passing through a semipermeable membrane.

cyanosis — a bluish-gray discoloration of the skin resulting from a deficiency of oxygen and an excess of carbon dioxide in the blood.

defibrillator — delivers electrical impulses to the heart, causing temporary cessation of cardiac activity, allowing time for the SA node to take over.

de Musset's sign — rhythmic shaking of the head due to pulsations of the carotid arteries; a sign of aortic insufficiency.

depolarization — equalization of ions on both sides of cell membrane with loss of electrical charge or polarity.

diastole — relaxation phase of cardiac cycle when ventricles are filling; between contractions.

Dressler's syndrome — postmyocardial infarction syndrome. A group of symptoms thought to result from antigen-antibody reaction and difficult to distinguish from extension or recurrence of an infarction.

dyskinesis — difficult or impaired expansion of part of the ventricular wall during systole.

echocardiography — ultrasonic waves directed through the chest wall transmitting and recording the position and motion of the heart and valves.

ectopic focus — in cardiology, a source of cardiac stimulus other than the SA node; usually caused by some irritation of the myocardium.

electrophoresis — a laboratory method used to analyze the plasma's protein content.

embolus — undissolved matter in the bloodstream; a traveling thrombus.

epicardium — outer covering of the heart; also called the visceral pericardium.

extrasystole — a premature contraction of the heart.

fibrillation — abnormal, rapid, chaotic arrhythmia of either atria or ventricles that prevents efficient myocardial contractility.

gallop rhythm — the occurrence of three or four extra heart sounds during diastole.

HDL — high-density lipoproteins; high levels in the blood serum indicate a decreased risk of coronary artery disease.

heart block — impaired impulse conduction of the heart; can occur any place in the heart; usually applied to atrioventricular heart block.

histamine — an amine, present in all body tissue; causes dilation of capillaries, increased gastric secretion, and constriction of bronchial smooth muscles.

holosystolic — refers to the entire systolic phase of the cardiac cycle.

Holter monitor — ambulatory electrocardiography; useful in diagnosing arrhythmias and causes of CNS symptoms, such as dizziness, syncope, and pain.

hyperlipidemia — abnormally high levels of lipids (fats) in the blood.

hyperpnea — a detectable increase in respiratory rate, above that normally seen in resting individuals.

hypertrophy — increased size of an organ or structure due to functional activity; not an increase in cells or tissue.

hypovolemia — abnormal decrease in blood volume.

(continued on next page)

ischemia — localized deficiency of blood caused by constriction or obstruction of the blood vessel to that area.

isoelectric — the baseline in an electrocardiogram.

millivolt — one-thousandth of a volt.

monitor — to watch continuously, observing and recording vital signs and other pertinent data; an apparatus used to observe and record physiological signs, for example, EKG, Holter monitor, etc.

mural — occurring in or referring to the wall of an organ or part. (For example: Mural thrombus occurs on the interior wall of the heart.)

murmur — sound heard upon auscultation of the heart. It is produced by vibrations caused by movement of blood in the heart and large vessels during systole or diastole.

myocardial catecholamines — group of neurohormones having an adrenergic effect on the heart.

myocardial infarction — tissue necrosis caused by myocardial ischemia.

myocardial insufficiency — weakening of the heart muscle that reduces the force whereby blood is ejected from the heart.

myocardial ischemia — a condition resulting from blood and oxygen starvation of the heart muscle.

myxoma, atrial — a benign gelatinous growth composed of primitive, mucous connective tissue.

nephrosclerosis — a hardening of the kidney due to renovascular disease.

neurohormones — hormones that stimulate neural responses.

orthopnea — difficulty breathing except in an upright position.

pacemaker — the SA node, so called because it initiates the electrical impulses that set the rhythm of cardiac contractions. An artificial pacemaker: an electrical device to pace cardiac rhythm.

palpitations — awareness of excessively rapid, fluttering heartbeats; may produce a high degree of anxiety.

papilledema —swelling of the optic disk; usually associated with intracranial pressure.

paradoxical pulse —fades away on inspiration and is weak on expiration because of changed intrathoracic pressures.

paroxysmal atrial tachycardia (PAT), paroxysmal supraventricular tachycardia (PSVT) — an arrhythmia characterized by the sudden onset of rapid, regular heartbeats in excess of 150 to 250 beats/minute.

pericardiocentesis — puncture of the sac around the heart for the purpose of withdrawing fluid.

pericardium — a fibroserous, fluid-filled sac surrounding the heart and the origins of the great vessels; composed of two layers, the visceral and the parietal.

peripheral vascular resistance — the force opposing the flow of blood through the vessels; depends on the size of the vessel and viscosity of fluid it contains.

petechiae — small, purplish, nonraised spots on the surface of the skin caused by intradermal or submucous hemorrhage.

pH — hydrogen ion concentration; denotes acidity or alkalinity of a solution; a pH over 7 means a solution is alkaline; under 7 means acid.

pheochromocytoma — a tumor of the adrenal medulla that causes hypertension by overproducing adrenal hormones.

phlebothrombosis — clotting in a vein unassociated with inflammation of the vessel walls.

phonocardiography — sounds of heart action recorded graphically on paper.

plaque — an accumulation of fatty material within the arterial intima.

pleura — moist lining of the chest wall that encloses the pleural cavity.

pneumothorax — air or gas in the pleural cavity that causes collapse of all or part of a lung.

premature ventricular contraction (PVC) — the most common ventricular arrhythmia, it occurs during diastole and originates from a focus somewhere in the ventricle. It may be normal or the result of irritation, ischemia, or drug therapy.

pulmonary wedge pressure (PWP) — measures left atrial pressure and left ventricular end-diastolic pressure (LVEDP) by means of a bulb-tipped catheter wedged in a small branch of the pulmonary artery; the most accurate means of predicting incipient heart failure.

pulse deficit — difference between apical and radial pulses when taken simultaneously.

pulsus alternans — strong beats alternating with weak beats while heart rhythm remains uninterrupted.

pulsus bisferiens — two arterial pulsations of almost equal strength per one heartbeat.

rales — abnormal respiratory sound heard on auscultation; may be dry or moist.

Raynaud's phenomenon — arterial spasms of the extremities precipitated by cold. They cause blanching, cold, and numbness followed by redness, warmth, and tingling.

repolarization — return to resting potential or polarity in the cell membrane.

retinopathy — generally any noninflammatory disease of the retina.

rheumatic heart disease — permanent damage to the heart, usually valvular, caused by recurrent attacks of rheumatic fever.

sarcoidosis — a chronic, progressive, generalized disorder that may affect any part of the body but especially lymph tissue; characterized by the presence of epithelioid cell tubercles that gradually change to fibrous tissue.

serum glutamic-oxaloacetic transaminase (SGOT) — an enzyme present in cardiac cells that escapes into the bloodstream upon tissue death and can be measured to assess damage.

sick sinus syndrome — alternating tachy- and bradyarrhythmia that appears in chronic ischemic heart disease when the SA node cannot respond correctly.

sinoatrial (SA) node — a small collection of neuromuscular tissue located near the junction of the superior vena cava and right atrium, which normally serves as the cardiac pacemaker.

stenosis — a narrowing or constricting of an opening.

Stokes-Adams syndrome — sudden attacks of unconsciousness, sometimes coupled with convulsions, which may accompany heart block or ventricular arrhythmia as a result of low cardiac output.

Swan-Ganz catheter — a flow-directed, balloon-tipped catheter inserted in a central venous position and advanced to the pulmonary artery; used to monitor pulmonary capillary or wedge pressure.

sympatholytics — agents that block the transmission of impulses from the adrenergic postganglionic fibers to effector organs or tissues inhibiting smooth-muscle contraction and glandular secretion.

systole — the contraction phase of the heart muscle that forces blood from the ventricles into the pulmonary artery and aorta.

tachycardia — heart rate usually greater than 100 beats/minute; it may be sinusal, atrial, junctional, or ventricular.

tachypnea — rapid, shallow breathing.

tamponade, cardiac — an accumulation of blood in the pericardial sac; it compresses the heart and inhibits diastolic filling; also called hemopericardium.

tetralogy of Fallot — congenital heart defect due to structural abnormalities. The cyanosis of infants born with this defect — referred to as blue babies — results from oxygenated blood from the lungs mixing with oxygen-depleted blood from the systemic circulation.

thoracentesis — surgical puncture of the thoracic cavity for the purpose of removing excess fluid.

thrombolytic agents — drugs that dissolve or break up clots.

thrombophlebitis — the development of clots in the presence of inflammatory changes in venous walls.

thrombus — a stationary clot in the circulatory system that frequently obstructs a vessel or cavity.

thrill — a very fine tremor felt on palpation, produced by a turbulent blood flow; also felt on palpation of aneurysm.

thyrotoxicosis — a thyroid disorder resulting from overproductivity of thyroid gland; characterized by accelerated pulse rate, exophthalmos, increased metabolic rate, and nervous symptoms.

triglyceride — a kind of lipid in the bloodstream; a glycerol bound to fatty acids.

Valsalva's maneuver — bearing down or forced exhalation effort against a closed glottis, which slows the heart rate.

varices — enlarged, tortuous abnormalities of the veins that may be caused by increased venous pressure and valvular weakness.

vasoconstrictor — See *vasopressor*.

vasodilator — an agent that relaxes (dilates) venous or arterial vessel walls.

vasopressor — an agent that stimulates generalized vasoconstriction, usually increasing blood flow to the body's vital organs.

vena cava — large vessel that returns blood to the heart: the superior drains from head and upper torso; the inferior, from the lower extremities and abdominal cavity.

ventricular escape — occurs when impulse conduction in the ventricular pacemaker fires before the impulse in the sinoatrial node.

ventriculography — visualization of the ventricles after introduction of a contrast medium.

COMMON CARDIOVASCULAR ABBREVIATIONS

AAA	—	abdominal aortic aneurysm
ABG	—	arterial blood gas
AMI	—	acute myocardial infarction
ASD	—	atrial septal defect
ASHD	—	arteriosclerotic heart disease
AV	—	atrioventricular
BPM	—	beats per minute
CAD	—	coronary artery disease
CCU	—	coronary care unit
CHF	—	congestive heart failure
COU	—	coronary observation unit
CPK	—	creatine phosphokinase
CPR	—	cardiopulmonary resuscitation
CVA	—	cerebrovascular accident
CVP	—	central venous pressure
EKG	—	electrocardiogram
HDL	—	high density lipoprotein
IAPB	—	intraaortic balloon pump
ICU	—	intensive care unit
IHSS	—	idiopathic hypertrophic subaortic stenosis
LAD	—	left anterior descending coronary artery
LAP	—	left atrial pressure
LC	—	left circumflex artery
LCA	—	left coronary artery
LDH	—	lactic dehydrogenase
LM	—	left main
LVEDP	—	left ventricular end-diastolic pressure
MCL	—	midclavicular line
PA	—	pulmonary artery
PAC	—	premature atrial contractions
PAP	—	pulmonary arterial pressure
PAT	—	paroxysmal atrial tachycardia
PCO_2	—	partial pressure of carbon dioxide
PDA	—	patent ductus arteriosus
PMI	—	point of maximal impulse
PO_2	—	partial pressure of oxygen
PSVT	—	paroxysmal supraventricular tachycardia
PTT	—	partial thromboplastin time
PVC	—	premature ventricular contraction
PWP	—	pulmonary wedge pressure
RCA	—	right coronary artery
RHD	—	rheumatic heart disease
SA	—	sinoatrial
SBE	—	subacute bacterial endocarditis
SGOT	—	serum glutamic-oxaloacetic transaminase
VSD	—	ventricular septal defect

Index

Page numbers followed by the letter "t" indicate both tabular and marginal material.

Selected References

Alpert, Joseph S., and Francis, Gary S. *Manual of Coronary Care,* 2nd ed. Boston: Little, Brown & Co., 1980.

Andreoli, Kathleen G., et al. *Comprehensive Cardiac Care: A Text for Nurses, Physicians and Other Health Practitioners,* 5th ed. St. Louis: C.V. Mosby Co., 1983.

Bavin, R. "Pediatric Cardiac Preoperative Teaching: A Family-Centered Approach," *Focus on Critical Care* 10:36-43, June 1983.

Chatterjee, K., et al. "Vasodilator Therapy for Heart Failure," *Critical Care Quarterly* 4:13-24, December 1981.

Cohen, M.A., "The Use of Prostaglandins and Prostaglandin Inhibitors in Critically Ill Neonates," *American Journal of Maternal Child Nursing* 8:194-199, May/June 1983.

Constant, Jules. *Bedside Cardiology,* 2nd ed. Boston: Little, Brown & Co., 1976.

Diagnostics. Nurse's Reference Library, Springhouse, Pa.: Springhouse Corp., 1981.

Diseases. Nurse's Reference Library. Springhouse, Pa.: Springhouse Corp., 1981.

Drugs. Nurse's Reference Library. Springhouse, Pa.: Springhouse Corp., 1982.

Ellestad, Myrin H. *Stress Testing: Principles and Practice.* Philadelphia: F.A. Davis Co., 1980.

Giving Cardiac Care. Nursing Photobook Series. Springhouse, Pa.: Springhouse Corp., 1981.

Haralambos, Gavras. "Hypertension and Congestive Heart Failure: Benefits of Converting Enzyme Inhibition Captopril," *Journal of the American College of Cardiology* 1:518-20, February 1983.

Harvey, A.M., ed. *The Principles and Practice of Medicine,* 20th ed. East Norwalk, Conn.: Appleton-Century-Crofts, 1980.

Hurst, J. Willis, and Logue, R. Bruce, eds. *The Heart,* 3rd ed. New York: McGraw-Hill Book Co., 1974.

Jones, Patricia. *Cardiac Pacing.* Myocardial Infarction Series. East Norwalk, Conn.: Appleton-Century-Crofts, 1980.

King, Ouida M. *Care of the Cardiac Surgical Patient.* St. Louis: C.V. Mosby Co., 1975.

Lowell, J.R. *Pleural Effusions: A Comprehensive Treatise.* Baltimore: University Park Press, 1976.

Meltzer, L.E., et al. *Intensive Coronary Care: A Manual for Nurses,* 3rd ed. Bowie, Md.: Charles Press Pubs., 1977.

Moss, Arthur J., et al, eds. *Heart Disease in Infants and Adolescents,* 2nd ed. Baltimore: Williams & Wilkins Co., 1977.

Perloff, Joseph. *Physical Examination of the Heart and Circulation.* Philadelphia: W.B. Saunders Co., 1982.

Ravin, A. *Ausculation of the Heart,* 3rd ed. Chicago: Year Book Medical Pubs., 1977.

Selzer, Arthur. *Principles of Clinical Cardiology.* Philadelphia: W.B. Saunders Co., 1975.

Stone, J. Gilbert, et al. "Sodium Nitroprusside Therapy for Cardiac Failure in Anesthesized Patients with Valvular Insufficiency," *Anesthesiology* 49:414-18, December 1978.

Sweetwood, Hannelore. *The Patient in the Coronary Care Unit.* New York: Springer Publishing Co., 1976.

Thompson, Donald A. *Cardiovascular Assessment: Guide for Nurses and Other Health Professionals.* St. Louis: C.V. Mosby Co., 1981.

Tucker, Susan M., et al. *Patient Care Standards,* 2nd ed. St. Louis: C.V. Mosby Co., 1980.

Vestal, Katherine W. *Pediatric Critical Care Nursing.* New York: John Wiley & Sons, 1981.

Whaley, Lucille F., and Wong, Donna L. *Nursing Care of Infants and Children,* 2nd ed. St. Louis: C.V. Mosby Co., 1983.

ACKNOWLEDGEMENTS

p. 18   Table and statistical information courtesy: Vaughan and McKay, *Textbook of Pediatrics,* Tenth edition. W.B. Saunders Company, 1975, p. 1003, 1098.

p. 29   Photos courtesy: *The Heart,* Fourth edition by Hurst et. al. Copyright 1978 by McGraw-Hill, Inc. Used with permission of McGraw-Hill Book Company.

p. 37   Photos courtesy: Public Relations Department, Children's Hospital of Philadelphia.

p. 56   X-ray courtesy: Peter G. Lavine, MD, Crozer-Chester Medical Center, Chester, Pa.

p. 64   Cines courtesy: Peter G. Lavine, MD.

p. 70   Photo courtesy: Temple University Department of Ophthalmology, Philadelphia.

p. 79   Coronary arteriogram courtesy: Marc S. Lapayowker, MD, Department of Radiology, Abington (Pa.) Memorial Hospital.

p. 96   X-ray courtesy, Peter G. Lavine, MD.

p. 111   Cine courtesy: Peter G. Lavine, MD.

p. 117   Photo courtesy: Gerald Pearlman, Skin and Cancer Hospital, Temple University Health Sciences Center, Philadelphia.

p. 120   X-ray courtesy: Peter G. Lavine, MD.

p. 129   Photos courtesy: Medical Monitors, Inc., Wyncote, Pa.

p. 139   Scans courtesy: John Reilley, Temple University Hospital, Department of Nuclear Medicine, Philadelphia.

p. 161   Photos courtesy: Moschella and Pillsbury, *Dermatology.* W.B. Saunders Company, 1975. Volume 1, p. 841.

p. 173   Rehab chart courtesy: Kathryn A. Hoffman, MD, Assistant Professor Rehabilitation Medicine, Emory University, Atlanta.